365

Ways to

Feel Better

'This book will transform your life. Radical self-care in easy baby steps, what's not to love?' ~ Suzy Greaves, Psychologies Editor and author of *Making the Big Leap*

'I am a great believer that we transform our lives through the cumulative effect of countless baby steps. Eve has done a remarkable job of pulling together 366 daily steps to help you live a happier, healthier, freer and more fulfilled life. Let her be your inspiring guide for your year.' ~ Nick Williams, best-selling author of fourteen books including *The Work We Were Born To Do* www.iamnickwilliams.com

'This is a fabulous book. So very well thought out, planned and executed and with a wonderful accessible yet respectful style. Buy yourself this book and sit down and devour it in the way that suits you best. Then buy a copy for someone else.' ~ Debra Jinks, co-author of *Personal Consultancy: A Model for Integrating Counselling and Coaching*

'It's hard to imagine a more useful book than the one you're holding in your hands. What Eve Menezes Cunningham has gathered here are easy to implement small changes that can keep you moving forward into greater well-being. Buy this book, make a note on your calendar that you're starting a new year of positive activity, do the first exercise. Then do the next one tomorrow. Simple as that. Keep it up and you'll be amazed at how far you've come after 365 days of taking small actions.' ~ Barbara J. Winter, author, *Making a Living Without a Job and Winning Ways newsletter*

'An interesting read which takes a range of theories, some traditional and some not, and applies them to the human condition. Written in an accessible style, a book that many will find of value.' ~ Gladeana McMahon, FAC, FBACP,FIMS, FIMS, FRSA, Chair Emeritus, Association for Coaching UK and author of books including *Resilience: A Practical Guide*

'Rich, extensive content covering a wide range of holistic principles and practices made very attainable for anyone to use. A wealth of options for managing being human.' ~ Gill Fennings-Monkman MBE, Past Chair of BACP Coaching

'I love how digestible the daily readings are. Motivational and not dictatorial. Love the language. Delicious.' ~ Ani Richardson, author of *Love or Diet: Nurture Yourself and Release the Need to be Comforted by Food*

'What a fabulous concept, 366 ways to feel better every day! If living a happy, loving and healthier life is of interest to you then pick up this book. Something here for everyone. Packed with inspiring ideas to get you off the sofa and deep into the possibilities of your life. Wish I had something like this a few years back.' ~ Steve Ahnael Nobel, author of *The Prosperity Game*

365

Ways to
Feel Better

Self-care Ideas for Embodied Wellbeing

EVE MENEZES CUNNINGHAM

*Original artwork and other illustrations by Amy Brennan-Whittington
and photos by Alan Cunningham*

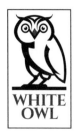

WHITE
OWL

First published in Great Britain in 2017 by
WHITE OWL
An imprint of
Pen & Sword Books Ltd
47 Church Street
Barnsley
South Yorkshire
S70 2AS

ISBN 978 1 47389 279 8

Typeset in Times New Roman by
CHIC GRAPHICS

Printed and bound in Malta
By Gutenberg Press Ltd.

Pen & Sword Books Ltd incorporates the Imprints of
Pen & Sword Archaeology, Atlas, Aviation, Battleground, Discovery,
Family History, History, Maritime, Military, Naval, Politics, Railways,
Select, Transport, True Crime, Fiction,
Frontline Books, Leo Cooper, Praetorian Press,
Seaforth Publishing, Wharncliffe and White Owl.

For a complete list of Pen & Sword titles please contact
PEN & SWORD BOOKS LIMITED
47 Church Street, Barnsley, South Yorkshire, S70 2AS, England
E-mail: enquiries@pen-and-sword.co.uk
Website: www.pen-and-sword.co.uk

Contents

To anyone who has ever felt broken beyond repair.
There is a part of you that is already whole.
More than whatever you've survived or struggle with.

Acknowledgements

As well as being grateful to *all* my clients, students, editors and readers, I appreciate every teacher and trainer and my fellow students.

Unless otherwise indicated:

- The psychosynthesis tools come from my training at the Psychosynthesis Education Trust at London Bridge. Thanks to all my trainers, supervisors and peers there, especially Brian Graham, Keith Sylvester, Duncan Lawrence, Pia Hoffman-Hansen, Claudia Carvalho, Joseph Allen, Lorna Clay, Ruth Dormandy, Derek Mutti and Allan Frater. And most of all, my training therapist, Lorraine Jury.

- The yoga, mindfulness and neuroscience related ideas come from my initial yoga therapy training with Heather Mason at the Minded Institute. Thanks, Heather, for creating this integrative model, for believing in my ability to grow into a yoga therapist and teacher when I didn't believe in myself and for your pioneering work in the field of yoga and mental health. Thanks also to the wonderful supervisors, especially Veena Ugargol and Elizabeth Bourdon

- NLP from my training up to Master Practitioner level with Bob Roberts and Annie Lennox of INLPTA.

- EFT from my training up to Advanced Practitioner level with Julia Johnson.

- Crystals from Stephanie Harrison who helped me kickstart my own healing process and changed my life.

Enormous thanks also to Joan Wilmot and Robin Shohet of CSTD London and Nash Popovic at the University of East London for the integrative counselling and coaching training (the first at post graduate level in this country). This helped me not only integrate the coach-therapy but to bring in my other therapies as appropriate, in a collaborative way.

Big appreciation to all my yoga teachers, especially Emma Turnbull, Allison Kelsey, Jean Hill and many from when I first started whose names I don't remember. All helped me (I know this sounds melodramatic) transform from being unable to stand upright due to chronic pain to being stronger, fitter and healthier than ever and able to share these tools with my clients, students and readers. And a special shout out to Ally for reminding me that sometimes, our yoga is a hot water bottle.

To my British Association for Counselling and Psychotherapy (BACP) Coaching Executive colleagues over the years, especially Gill Fennings-Monkman MBE, Steve Page, Carolyn Mumby, Michèle Down and Sally Brown.

And to my freelance friends (some of whom I still only 'know' online) thanks for more support, encouragement and inspiration over the years than you probably realise.

Enormous thanks to the friends and colleagues who read sections and drafts in advance, encouraging me and helping me to improve it. Especially Alexandra Maeja Raicar, Steve Page, Michèle Down, Bev Bennett Boss, Gill Fennings-Monkman, Suzy Greaves, Jemma Prittie, Claudia Cahalane, Mike Smallpage, Amy Brennan-Whittington, Ani Richardson, Emma Turnbull, Imogen Goodchild and Claire Jaques. Thanks also to Jan Cadman.

Thanks to Kate Bohdanowicz, Carol Trow and all at White Owl (at Pen & Sword publishing), especially Jonathan Wright, Lori Jones, Heather Williams, Lauren Burton and Jodie Butterwood.

Additional thanks to Amy Brennan-Whittington for the illustrations and Jon Wilkinson for the cover design. Luke Magnay at Cloud Media for the bonus videos and Kathie Bishop for too much to mention here.

To friends and family not mentioned above. Especially my father, Tim Cunningham, my brother, Alan Cunningham (for the photos and support) and, again, Claire Jaques.

And most of all, thanks to my mother, Alexandra Maeja Raicar.

Please read the following carefully:

Introduction

365 days, 366 ways to help yourself *Feel Better Every Day* – there's a bonus for leap years. This is to offer options. It's far from a definitive list of self-care ideas. There are so many things we can do to support ourselves, it was challenging narrowing them down to my top 366.

You might choose to read each day according to the calendar. The dates are in UK format (day/month). These dates in brackets are to lead you to other days which may help you with some more information. Alternatively, you could ask that wisest part of yourself for guidance, choosing one at random or from the Contents.

You might also simply like to jot down the titles of favourite tips (not just from this book but from the wider world and things that have worked for you in the past). Pop them on separate pieces of paper in a pretty vase, bag or box. Then, any time you need a boost, you don't need to stress yourself out by trying to consciously think of the best tool to play with; instead, you might ask to be guided to the right tip for that moment or open the book at random.

If you've been to a yoga class, you might be familiar with the idea of setting an intention for your practice. Increasingly, I encourage clients to do this at the start of every type of session I offer. To sit quietly, settle, tune into the natural breath and feel the earth's support. To think about what they most want to get out of the session. It only takes a few moments yet can bring a great deal of focus. You can use this same approach before choosing a tool for any day. What are your intentions for today? For this month? This year?

For the yoga tips, if you're new to yoga and don't know how to do these poses, please see a yoga therapist or instructor. If you're new to exercise, please consult your GP. Above all else, honour your body's own wisdom; you'll know which ideas feel good to you and which, for whatever reason, give you pause.

In Neuro Linguistic Programming (NLP), we talk about 'well-formed outcomes'. Taking a few moments before opening this book can help with this. Similarly, you're allowing yourself to be mindful of whatever happens to be going on for you; while it's called *Feel Better Every Day*, sometimes we just need permission to wallow and honour however we're feeling.

You're creating a space to allow your inner wisdom to come through. You may want to add qualities to your intentions, like love or grace. You may even want to add goals. By noticing whatever arises, you can choose a page to support you with that whenever you feel ready.

Some of the tools will appeal more than others. Feel free to explore these in more depth than I can go into here. I have included books, websites and other resources to help you do this. I've created some bonus videos for the yoga poses, breath practices, meditations and Emotional Freedom Techniques (EFT). These are available at www.feelbettereveryday.co.uk/book

I'm also aware that inclusive as I want to be, men may find some of the ideas less relevant – although they may help you better get to know and support the women in your lives. For these days – or *any* days that don't appeal – you might want to open the book at random for another tip.

Overall, I hope these tips will support you in making little tweaks to your life, creating new habits and helping yourself feel better every day. I also hope they'll remind you of all the things you already *know* help you feel better every day and that you'll make time for all of these supportive practices.

Social media: If you enjoy Facebook, you can find me at www.facebook.com/feelbettereveryday. I've created a group for readers to connect with me (I'll check in regularly to answer as many questions as possible) and each other and share how you're doing. You can join from within Facebook by searching *365 Ways to Feel Better: Self care Ideas for Embodied Wellbeing*.

You can also find me on twitter @wellbeingeve and Instagram @evemenezescunningham. Using the hashtag #365waystofeelbetter will help me see as many posts as possible.

I look forward to 'meeting' you.

January

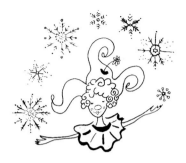

New Year, New You.

Do other people want to just crawl back under the duvet when reading such headlines?

This month's tips include exploring ways to start the year in ways that can support us in feeling better. These include a way to breathe more joy into your life. We're also looking at ways to open our hearts and remove possible resistance to even the idea of doing things differently.

1/1 - The Relaxation Response - treating our system to a New Year reboot

Back in 1975, Dr Herbert Benson, a cardiologist at Harvard, was sneaking Transcendental Meditators into his lab at night. They wanted him to study the effects of meditation on their hearts but he was embarrassed about what his colleagues might think. His risk paid off and, in the very same lab that Walter B. Cannon had discovered the fight/flight response **(3/4)** decades earlier, Benson discovered what he called the Relaxation Response.

This deep state of relaxation allows the body to recharge and heal at a greater rate than even during deep sleep. And it only takes a few minutes. While there are many meditative and relaxation techniques from around the world which help us enter this natural state, it doesn't have to be complicated.

Dr Benson, now in his 90s, continues to lecture around the world on mind-body medicine and recommends simply choosing a quality. Love? Grace? Peace? Joy? What springs to mind for you.

When I was taught this, I worried I had to commit to the one quality for each time I practiced it – not a thought process that was conducive to relaxation. Fortunately, we can even change it if needed within the three minute meditation. There's no need to overthink anything.

Sitting or lying comfortably, just inhale that quality … then exhale that quality.

Benson found that the Relaxation Response could be entered in as little as three minutes of doing this. Allowing ourselves a little longer can help us to relax into it. Even we only have a minute, it can still bring calming benefits. We're human. Our minds will wander. When we notice this happening, we can simply choose to bring our attention back to our breath and chosen quality.

Inhale (breathe it in) and exhale (breathe it out)…

You may want to read his book (*The Relaxation Response) *and check out* http://www.relaxationresponse.org/ *for more information

2/1 – *Next* New Year – what do you want to be different?

'*Next* New Year? Only just made it through this one,' you might be thinking, but taking this approach can help us focus.

Picture yourself having had a year that surpassed your wildest dreams for yourself. What kind of year, in this ideal world, has it been? How about when you think about your relationships? What were those highlights?

Maybe you met someone you feel great about? Maybe you ended a relationship that was way past its sell-by date. Maybe you opened up to your existing partner and improved your relationship. Maybe you started truly enjoying being alone.

While your ideal world highlights a year from now are clean and glossy, in reality, any of these options might have been messy: 'Will s/he ever call?'; 'What have I done?'; 'Urgh, this is the best I can hope to do?'; 'Are we opening an enormous can of worms by actually talking about our lives together?'

Whether you've been together a day or fifty years, making yourself vulnerable can be scary. As you imagine yourself a year from now, does the risk you imagined yourself taking feel worth it? From that Future You vantage point, is there anything else you would like to add? Think of it as breadcrumb trails to make it easier for Current You?

We can do the same with other areas of our lives, imagining our ideal world in terms of fun, money, home, work, big dreams, your spirit, home, travel, family, friends, health and fitness and any other categories you choose to add for yourself. How might each area of your life look a year from now? Which areas of your life stand out in terms of greatest imaginary improvement? At this point, be patient with yourself.

Let yourself picture everything being better than you've ever dreamed. You might want to make notes or sketches to represent what you can see, feel, hear, touch and even maybe taste from this 'wonderful life' as you live the Future You. You might even create a mood box (8/12).

Bringing it back to the present, take each area in turn. Ask yourself what steps you might start taking today in order to make as much of your ideal world a reality as you choose.

17/11 gives more ideas for deepening changes you may want to make.

3/1 – Setting your space

As part of my morning meditation, I include this visualisation from Art Giser, creator of Energetic NLP (ENLP). I set the space at home and for every space I'll be working in. It's especially helpful for my yoga classes, talks and workshops.

Picture a ball of universal energies in the centre of your home or whatever room you're in. Imagine it swirling happily, sending rays to each of the corners of the ceilings and floors. Visualise the ceilings, walls and floors being filled with this glorious universal energy.

Now imagine giant magnets above you, below, to the right and left, front and back. Let each magnet gently clear whatever energies are ready to be released from your energy field. They release all energies that aren't authentically yours, letting them be recycled to nourish the earth.

Let the magnets and any residual energies be taken for recycling by the earth. Imagine a ball of golden light, filled with your highest energies, about three feet above your head. Allow this light to draw back any energies you may have scattered and send rays of this light to the top and bottom corners of your energy field.

Fill the imaginary ceiling, walls and floor of your energy field (I imagine mine as a bubble) with this glorious, grounded golden light and bask in its radiance. Absorb as much of this light as possible, especially imagining it permeating areas where energies were released. You can repeat the process with your workspace, a meeting room, family dinner or anywhere you're going to be and would like a little more support.

You can imagine golden balls of light bouncing ahead of you easing travel and communications. And you can fill the spaces you're setting with as many healing energies as you want.

Giser encourages creativity **(6/6)** so if magnets don't do it for you, experiment with a vacuum cleaner or any other kind of cleaning equipment. Gently draw away stagnant energies that you're ready to be freed from. Remember to replace whatever you've released with that glorious golden, grounded light energy, setting your space and helping you flourish.

Find out more about working with your Miraculous Self and ENLP at www. energeticnlp.com and www.solar-events.co.uk for Art's courses and workshops in the UK.

4/1 – Setting intentions

This simple tool can be incredibly powerful. You can do it each day or for a yoga class or therapeutic session, party, interview or meeting.

Simply pause before any activity. How do you hope to feel afterwards? What do you want to achieve? This can help you work collaboratively while also lifting the energy of any group (and your own). Depending on the kind of meeting, you may find sharing your intention adds to the benefits. This won't always be appropriate. You know best.

Choosing an angel card* or similar can help. Sometimes, you might draw a card to embody that day and think, 'Absolutely! Spot on!' Other times, when feeling less focused while choosing, it may make no sense. This, too, is useful information and, of course, you can always choose another one. For example, whenever I draw Patience, I pick another for extra support in becoming more patient.

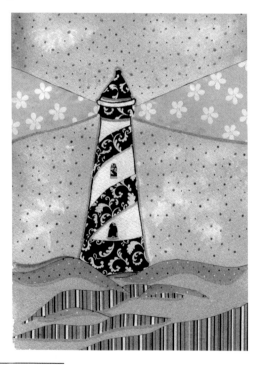

* I have several decks and especially love the simplicity of Joy Drake and Kathy Tyler's. They are available online and at many metaphysical gift shops. I also love Stephanie Harrison's online card reading app available for Android and Apple at www.lifeguidanceandinspiration.com

5/1 – Symbols

When I do my space clearing each morning **(5/3, 18/7, 29/7, 4/12)**, I add symbols to my home and work spaces. These include crystals **(22/8)**. For example, I often use imaginary obsidian **(2/9)** in the far corners for grounding and protection. I add whatever feels most appropriate for the day ahead. Clear quartz **(31/8)** for clarity, blue lace agate **(5/9)** for gentleness and amethyst **(29/8)** for wisdom and inspiration are current favourites. I sometimes include words and other symbols to help me focus on how I want to feel.

Incorporating these symbols (for example, a screenshot of a vision board, **(24/12)** or mantra, using your passwords as reminders) into our daily lives helps us keep them in mind, making them even more practical and powerful.

6/1 – Feeling blue?

The first working Monday of the year is known, in the UK, as Blue Monday. Fortunately, there are all sorts of ways we can lift our moods.

Moving and breathing differently changes the signals going from body to brain **(29/2)** and changes the way we feel more effectively, often, than simply trying to *tell* ourselves to feel something different.

Amy Weintraub, author of *Yoga for Depression* (Broadway Books, 2004), created the Breath of Joy to help us use our bodies to cheer ourselves up. Standing up, take three breaths in, moving your arms as if conducting an orchestra. Fold forward as you exhale with a 'Ha' and repeat a few rounds. Imagine inhaling joy and releasing whatever's keeping you stuck. After a few rounds, having got the prana (life energy) moving, pause and notice how you feel.

You can see Amy teach it at https://www.youtube.com/watch?vm=OZ3v3 w1h0g

7/1 – Mindful breathing

My yoga therapy training taught me that mindfulness of the breath is an easier place to start than mindfulness of the body or of thoughts. We tend to be more judgmental of our bodies and, initially, thoughts often move too quickly to be mindful of.

We have our breath with us 24/7 so it's a great tool in terms of regular practice. Even so, compassion **(22/12)** is a key component of mindfulness. It's not about, 'Urgh, what's *wrong* with me? I can't even *breathe* properly!'

Pause to notice the natural breath. If comfortable to do so, we can change it to one of the techniques outlined, like Ujjayi **(6/4)**, regulating our breath and improving our moods. These tips are *not* to stress you out. You're alive. You're breathing *fine*.

Still, conscious breathing has a whole host of benefits. With practice, we can use our breath to retrain the autonomic nervous system (ANS), strengthen the prefrontal cortex (which boosts concentration and emotional regulation) and reap the specific benefits of different breath practices. They don't require special equipment.

8/1 – Belly breath

Remember the story about the centipede? Asked how she managed to co-ordinate all those feet she suddenly couldn't do it and toppled over. Our breath can be similarly confusing when we start paying attention to it. Having something to focus on can help. Start by noticing, in a curious but non judgmental way, whether you're breathing from the top of the lungs, middle of the lungs or lower lungs, as if you were breathing from the belly.

Do you get a sense of where your natural breath is in this moment? Typically, when we're stressed or exercising, our breath is shallow. Often, we can consciously choose to bring our breath down as if from our belly. Do you immediately notice some calming benefits?

How does it feel to spend a few moments consciously breathing from the lower lungs right now?

For most people, abdominal breathing takes some concentration. This helps us stay more mindful of it. And, of course, when our minds *do* wander – we're human – we can bring our awareness back to our breath.

9/1 – Longer exhalation

Do you feel more comfortable with the idea of training your breath by breathing from the lower lungs **(8/1)**? Now take a moment to notice whether your inhalation is longer than your exhalation, if they're evenly balanced or if your exhalation is longer than your inhalation.

In terms of what's happening with our nervous systems, a longer inhalation (in other words, the sometimes misguided suggestion to 'take a deep breath and calm down') lifts the nervous system by activating the sympathetic branch of the nervous system. Lifting means activating the sympathetic branch while lowering is activating the parasympathetic branch and downgrading the stress response. An equal inhalation and exhalation balances the Autonomic Nervous System **(26/1)**. And a longer exhalation activates the parasympathetic branch (responsible for the rest/digest response **(1/1)**).

Our 24/7 society tends to mean it's lifted far more than our ancient ancestors experienced. This can be through busy lifestyles but even when we're not obviously doing something, we're often worrying about things and this lifts the nervous system, too. Choosing a longer exhalation when we're breathing mindfully helps balance the nervous system overall.

10/1 – What drives you?

Subpersonalities are a key concept in psychosynthesis. Nothing to be scared of, we *all* have them. When we observe them with curiosity and compassion, we're less likely to act out on them unconsciously. We are better able to become more whole. We might imagine the Self (that wise, observer aspect of ourselves) as Duke Ellington with our various subpersonalities as members of his big band. All the musicians are amazing but they need that strong bandleader to help them shine without any instruments taking over, causing musical mayhem.

Sometimes, we become aware of various subpersonalities (for example, our Anxious part, our Vulnerable part, our Angry part) and try to get rid of them. Yet no matter how irritating, they've helped us get through whatever stage of life brought them to the fore. We're much better off learning from them and integrating them. The following days **(11/1 - 19/1)**, though it's far from a definitive list, give some ideas how.

11/1 – Please yourself

The one time I hitch hiked, as a teenager, I was so relieved to not be murdered, I nearly invited the driver in for coffee. My Pleaser subpersonality used to run my life. It's easy to see how our Pleasers become so ingrained. When we're teeny tiny humans, dependent on adult carers with their own stresses, pleasing those adults (smiling, gurgling and doing what they want even when it doesn't feel good for us) enhances our chances for survival.

By adulthood, our Pleaser (like so many of our subpersonalities) is no longer so useful. By recognising those times it pops up (those times we say 'Yes' rather than 'No way', when we smile sweetly instead of allowing our face to rest in whichever expression feels best in the moment), we can become more aware of those times in our lives when we're giving our power away.

As with everything, it's a practice. The more ingrained, the more we need to be patient with ourselves. Sometimes we may notice our Pleaser and still choose to act on it. At least we're being more conscious of it.

When does your Pleaser pop up most?

12/1 – Rebel without a cause?

Does your inner Rebel get you into trouble? This is another common subpersonality which, again, would have been incredibly useful for us when younger and being endlessly told what we could and couldn't do. Having a strong Pleaser doesn't mean we don't also have a strong Rebel. The more we can integrate, rather than repressing less appreciated aspects, the more harmonious our lives can be.

Maybe your Rebel was your friend as a teenager but now gets you in trouble at work? Maybe you can call on your inner Rebel *more* in order to figure out how to get things done when others don't see a way forward? What springs to mind for you when you contemplate your inner Rebel?

What does it need from you? If you honour it enough to listen even for a moment, what gift is your inner Rebel offering you?

How can you listen so you're guided by it to improve your life rather than unconsciously acting out and potentially sabotaging yourself?

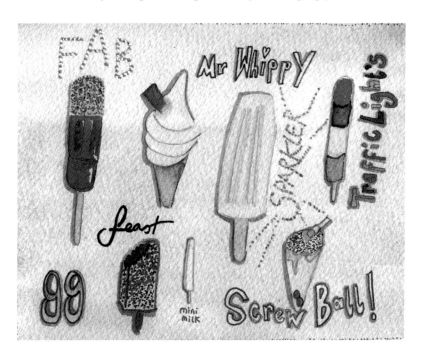

13/1 – Family ties

Some of our subpersonalities tie in with roles we occupy within our families. The clearer we can get on how all of these roles are just parts of us – that we are much more than just a mother, father, wife, husband, partner, son, daughter, sister, brother and so on - the easier it can become to balance family with work and the rest of our lives. When we over-identify with certain roles (especially if, for example, we had to become caregivers early on), it can be especially distressing when something happens to affect this important element of our identity (such as a break-up or bereavement).

Who are you as a mother, father, son, daughter, sister, brother or partner? What does this subpersonality need from you? How is it trying to help you? This can help you remember that there's more to you than this.

14/1 – Rescuer

Do you always have an eye out for someone in potential peril? Are you often more attuned to others' needs than to your own? My Rescuer subpersonality was one of my most entrenched and my counselling training eventually taught me to dial it back, to pause rather than leaping in trying to fix things.

Being human, it still surfaces sometimes but I've learned to be friendlier towards it. How is it trying to help me?

Getting to know our different subpersonalities doesn't mean eradicating anything. Having more awareness around them helps us use them more consciously rather than acting out unconsciously.

If you're a parent of a small child or responsible for an animal, obviously, continue caring appropriately. But when out with friends and grown adult relatives (or strangers), we can notice the impulse to help, rescue and fix.

When is your Rescuer useful? When might it be less so?

15/1 – Clowning around

Do you have a tendency to crack a joke at the first sign of trouble, unconsciously using humour to create a sense of safety?

As with all subpersonalities, our Clowns have a lot going for them. We're not aiming for sense of humour bypasses. When does it come from a full, safe, joyful place? When, perhaps, is it putting ourselves or others down in an effort to feel more connected by selling ourselves or others short?

What kind of jokes, comedies and situations bring out your happiest self? When does your Clown feel joyful? When might it be worth paying attention to in order to see what's going on behind that smile and what you really need right now?

16/1 – Victim

Ahhh, our Victim! So helpless; so blameless; so seductive! When do you notice yourself being most likely to forget your personal power and instead curl up in a ball and wait for life to kick you a bit more?

Terrible things happen. With legal situations, keeping people in victim mode can make their testimony better for the case. Even so, holding the awareness that we are more than whatever has happened, makes us less likely to forget our resources **(15/10)**.

This isn't letting anyone off the hook, simply remembering that we have survived. We have come through it. It was tough but we can do more of the things that nourish us.

When our resilience has been knocked, we're more likely to slip back into Victim roles. Obviously, we're not wanting to *blame* our Victims or make ourselves feel bad for having human responses to painful situations, but we can notice when we're slipping into powerlessness.

What does your Victim subpersonality need from you? Sometimes *our own* acknowledgment of the situation can be enough to help us move on. As with everything, it's a matter of practice.

17/1 – Inner queen or king

This isn't about being a diva or entitled in anyway. Instead, we're drawing on that spark we all have. The more we step into our power, the bigger the impact we can have in the world. Ask yourself what would your inner Queen (or King) do? To cook for lunch? When to spend (or save)? When would it be appropriate for them to turn up in your life and work?

Notice the different choices you make when your inner Queen or King is ruling and when you're acting from a less empowered subpersonality. Which do you prefer?

What does your inner Queen or King need from you in order to live more regally? This is about putting ourselves in a position to lift those around us up, too.

18/1 – Career related sub

When you imagine yourself without your job title, how do you feel? For some of us, it's challenging to imagine that being taken away somehow, through redundancy, retirement, parental leave and so on. For others, it has less impact. It depends on how much we identify with our work roles. As with all of our subpersonalities, we're looking at ways to expand our awareness around them. We can choose instead of feeling trapped.

When you fully identify with your work role, how do you feel? What are the benefits? Any blocks? What about if it were gone tomorrow? Would you still be getting dressed for work and leaving as if you were going there or would you happily throw yourself into new adventures?

How is your career subpersonality helping you? What does that aspect need from you? How can you start to enjoy more freedom around it?

19/1 – Embodying a subpersonality

Pick a sub, any sub **(10/1)**. It may be one of the ones mentioned above, or something else that springs to mind for you. The part of you that wants to change the world? Your Saboteur? Trust your inner wisdom.

Notice how you want to stand (or sit, or curl up in a ball) when you embody a particular subpersonality. Shake it off and pick another. How do you want to position yourself when you're tuned into this aspect of yourself? What have you learned about which subpersonalities feel comfortable and familiar but which may be holding you back?

Before shaking it off and choosing a more empowered one to embody, pause to ask each one, 'What do you need from me?' Remember that we are much more than each of these aspects and yet they've all developed as a survival mechanism. While probably inappropriate for our current lives, we benefit more by thanking them and figuring out healthier ways to meet those still important needs now rather than simply trying to kick them to the kerb.

Debbie Ford's **The Dark Side of the Light Chasers** *(Hodder, 2001) explores subpersonalities in more depth.*

20/1 – Timeline therapy

Developed by Tad James, this involves noting where you imagine your future in relationship to yourself – maybe pointing in front of you - and your past - maybe behind. These are common ones but we're all different, so tune into your own timeline and imagine it as one big timeline.

From this imaginary line, which we can highlight with pieces of paper or other markers, we can revisit past and future events from an empowered, resourceful state. We can shift our relationship to these events, for example, feeling more excited about an upcoming presentation.

The first time I did this, my entire past was like a bombsite. I was clinging onto the present and the future was fine. Over time, pieces of my past healed and became more visible. I even recovered more positive memories from those times. Like so many of these self-care ideas, it sounds a bit odd but can make a big difference.

timelinetherapy.com **gives more information.**

21/1 – Healing your whole timeline

Whether you're using a timeline and markers or simply taking old photos (and possibly creating future ones through aging apps) of yourself at different stages, the possibilities are endless. You might want to take a picture (or another marker for yourself at that age) and send Metta **(15/2)**, love and healing to that younger (or older) you. Be gentle with yourself. This kind of exercise is best done gradually and kindly rather than trying to force yourself before you feel ready.

If specific pictures bring up too much charge **(6/2)**, simply start by sending general love and healing energies down along the whole timeline going back to your past (maybe even back to before you were born) and way into your future.

As with all of these ideas, you know yourself best. Go with the ones that feel right for you at any given time.

22/1 – Chanting

Chanting has many benefits. Yes, you may feel a little embarrassed at first but you'll be surprised by how quickly loved ones and pets stop paying the slightest attention. Like singing **(2/3)**, chanting naturally elongates the exhalation **(9/1)** so helps activate the parasympathetic, calming branch of the autonomic nervous system.

It's a mindfulness tool, too. Sometimes, our voices are clear and strong, indicating balanced throat chakras (13/7). Other days, they may be weaker and more hesitant. Noticing this during a morning meditative practice means we can take extra steps to be extra gentle with ourselves throughout the day.

You might want to simply chant a simple mantra like Om (Ahh, Uuhhh, Mmm). I'll introduce additional options in the following days (23/1, 17/7).

A 2011 study found that chanting Om reduced limbic activation (including in the right amygdala which is often activated during emotional turmoil) and Telles' 1995 research found it slowed the heart rate. Chanting helps improve lung capacity as well as helping us access meditative states.

How do you feel when you chant Om?

23/1 – Open your heart with Om Mani Padme Hum

One of my favourite mantras to chant is Om Mani Padme Hum. I learned it on my initial yoga therapy training and it means, 'My heart is opening like the jewel in a lotus blossom'.

On days when we feel comfortable encouraging our hearts to open more, it's a beautiful practice.

While traditionally done in a comfortable seated position (either on the floor or on a chair, with the spine as straight as feels comfortable), I often teach it in Restorative Fish pose (11/2) as this supports the heart opening from a supported place. Play with your favourite positions.

24/1 - Yoga strap for heart opening

A simple way to open your heart centre is to take a yoga strap (if you don't have one, any belt or scarf will be fine) and play. Starting with the hands

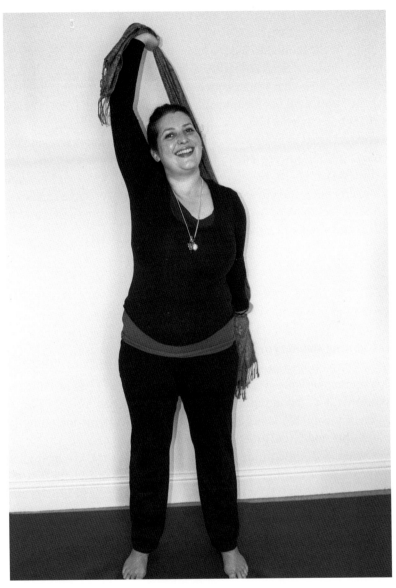

holding it about shoulder distance apart, above the head, allow yourself to use the strap's resistance to stretch yourself as needed.

Play with different degrees of intensity as you gently take the strap in front, behind and around the upper body. Hold your hands further apart or closer together depending on what feels best for you.

25/1 - *Santes Dwynwen* and the heart chakra

Although I'll talk about the chakras later (**9/7 to 17/7**), the Welsh equivalent of Saint Valentine's feast day feels like a nice day to introduce the heart chakra (**12/7**). When our heart centres are in balance, we're able to give and receive love with ease. As the middle of the main seven chakras, a balanced heart chakra can help us integrate, balancing the whole system.

You might want to bring your awareness to your heart centre and notice any charge (**6/2**). If it were able to talk to you, what might it tell you it needs more (or less) of?

Is it overly open and vulnerable? Maybe it's overly protected and closed? How does it feel to place both hands over the heart centre (in the middle of the chest) and simply breathe in and out?

26/1– Calming the nervous system

The autonomic nervous system (ANS) helps us do all sorts of things (like breathing) without having to think about it. As a bonus, when we do such things consciously, the benefits affect our whole systems including heart rate variability and blood pressure.

Practising tools that move us from sympathetic (fight/flight) to parasympathetic (rest/digest, including the even deeper benefits of the Relaxation Response (**1/1**)) mean that even when life gets hectic, we can be more resilient.

For example, I was in an odd situation recently where a troubled young man was swearing at me, incessantly, as I attempted to read peacefully.

It took me a very long time to read one paragraph as I was so shocked by this but not in a position to leave; in other words, I couldn't honour my natural flight impulse. Years of doing this work and practicing these tools, especially the breath and bodywork, meant that when I was safely away, it didn't take long to return to a calmer state. Over the years, I have improved my autonomic resilience.

As I felt better, I realised that instead of failing to read that same paragraph

18

over and over, I *could* have put the book down and focused on my Ujayyi breathing **(6/4)** to activate the parasympathetic branch **(9/1)**. In reality, I did the best I could in the situation. Through regular practice, I was able to use some self-soothing tools soon enough. If I am ever in a similar situation, I can see (if it feels safe enough) if Ujjayi feels appropriate in that moment.

27/1 – Bedtime pictures

Sleep expert Philip Stevens/Swami Sannyasananda suggests moving from the more intellectual, wordy way of thinking we typically live in to a gentler, more visual state before bedtime. This might be where the idea of counting sheep came from. Visualising helps us prepare ourselves for a good night's sleep and can also help us have more pleasant dreams **(5/7)**.

Before you go to sleep, you can quiet the mind by imagining something really pleasant. You might take yourself to your Happy Place **(17/12)** or visualise tomorrow going better than you might even imagine.

We regularly unconsciously catastrophise, imagining all sorts of horrors in graphic detail. This tends to keep us awake. By choosing something more pleasant to ponder, we remind ourselves to make necessary changes in our waking life as well as improving our sleep.

28/1 – Yogic twists to help us digest life

When our digestion is working well, we're better able to relax and sleep. Holding yogic twists for three minutes or longer can aid digestion.

These twists **(29/1-1/2)** impact different parts of the torso and internal organs to varying degrees. As with all yoga poses, we don't have to look like the model yogis on Instagram to benefit our own bodies and minds.
I hope you'll enjoy experimenting with these twists over the next few days.

29/1 – Supine spinal twist

This is one of my favourites. It can even be done in bed.

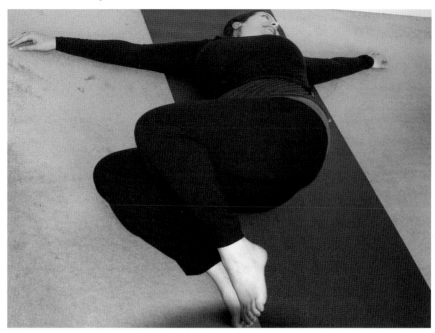

- ✓ Lying on your mat with the back with your head, neck and spine nicely aligned, take the arms out to the sides so you're forming a T shape with your torso and arms.

- ✓ Bending your knees, bring the soles of the feet to the floor. You can have the knees raised, parallel to the hips with the calves parallel to the floor if you want a deeper twist.

- ✓ Keeping both shoulder blades grounded, turn the head to look over the right shoulder as you allow the knees to fall towards the left side.

- ✓ Notice what happens to your breath and aim to keep it steady, breathing as if from the belly, with a longer exhalation.

- ✓ You might want to take just a few (five) complete breaths here or, time three minutes.

✓ Bring the head and knees back to the centre.

✓ Pause to notice how both sides feel in comparison to each other.

✓ Repeat on the other side.

30/1 – Simple twist

✓ Sitting cross legged (if this isn't comfortable, sit with both legs outstretched in front of you), take the left hand onto the right knee (or if legs are outstretched, onto the right thigh) and turn your head to look over your right shoulder.

✓ Again, notice what happens to your breath. Aim to keep it steady, deep, as if breathing from your belly, with a longer, calming exhalation.

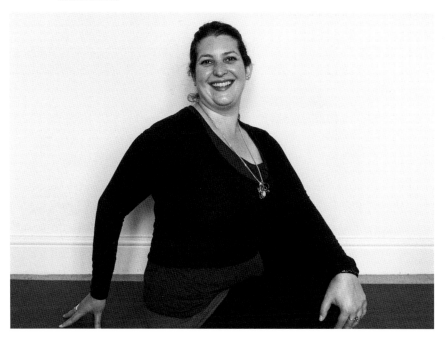

- ✓ After a few (five if that feels good) complete breaths here (or at least three minutes for those digestive benefits), turn your head back to the centre and bring both hands back to your knees or lap.

- ✓ Pause to notice how both sides feel before repeating on the other side.

31/1 – Seated twist

This is great for offering our bodies a deeper detoxifying twist and learning to control the breath. Keeping the breath deep, with that calming exhalation **(9/1)** here, in a more dynamic pose, means we're better able to calm ourselves and digest life off the yoga mat, too.

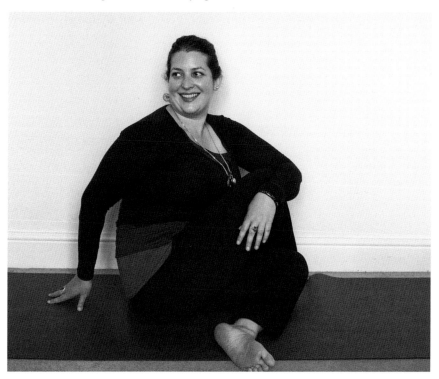

- ✓ Sitting with your legs in front of you, take the left foot over the right knee.

- ✓ Hug the inside of the left knee with the inside of the right elbow and turn to look over the left shoulder.

- ✓ Hold for a few complete breaths (five if that feels good or at least three minutes for extra digestive benefits) before turning your head back.

- ✓ Release the right arm and left leg, pausing to notice how both sides feel and repeating on the other side.

February

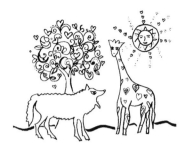

This month's tips include more heart opening practices, new growth in our lives (and supporting ourselves through it), talking to ourselves more kindly (so we stop ripping ourselves to shreds with our thoughts), and tuning into our inner wisdom more.

1/2 – Triangle pose

This is a great way to train the whole vestibular system for mental and physical balance. It helps strengthen our base chakra **(9/7)** as well as being a lovely heart opener **(9/2)**.

Staying grounded, we can open our hearts as we reach for the heavens. Triangle is both lifting and grounding.

- ✓ Start by standing with the right foot facing the short end of the mat and the left foot facing the long end, with both heels parallel to the mat. This can be used as a guideline.
- ✓ Bring the arms up to shoulder height. Elongate through the right side of the body so you start feeling your left side of the torso. Bring the right hand down onto the right leg or floor, wherever feels best.
- ✓ This is about keeping the heart centre open so roll the left shoulder back and bring the left hand higher up the right leg to keep this expansive heart. Can you feel it in the left side of the torso? Keep the torso straight and the left side long.
- ✓ Lift the left arm up and, if comfortable for your neck, look up at it. If not, look at the floor. As with all yoga poses, pay more attention to your own body's wisdom than anything else.

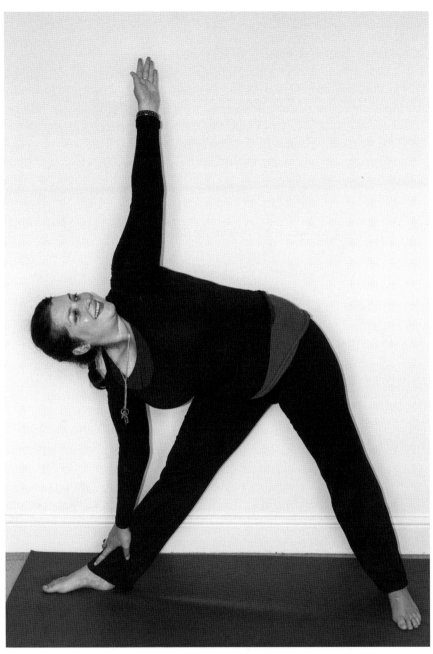

✓ Triangle allows full thoracic breathing **(3/2)**. Stay for a few complete breaths (maybe five if that feels good) here before gently coming back up to standing, pausing to notice how each side feels. Repeat on the left.

2/2 – Happy Imbolc/Brigid! – Defrosting our dreams

This is all about renewal. Spring hasn't reached the UK but we're generally starting to crave that warmth, imagining what we'll do when the sun returns. A simple way to honour this feast is to turn on all the lights in your home for a few minutes, symbolically welcoming the sun back in.

It's also a great time to think about the light within, how we want to shine in the world and what we're ready to contribute. With all your lights blazing, give yourself permission to dream big. What would you do if you weren't afraid to shine?

How can you connect with your inner light more?

3/2 – Three-part breath

There are many, many types of pranayama (yogic breath practices). This is a simple one you can play with to better acquaint yourself with your lungs.

- ✓ Lying or sitting down (lying down might be easier), start by resting the hands on your belly. Bring your awareness to each inhalation and exhalation as your abdomen rises and falls with every breath.
- ✓ When you feel ready (maybe after five breaths with this focus), bring your hands to your floating ribs, so you're holding the thumbs and index fingers around your side at approximately the level of a woman's bra strap at the sides.
- ✓ This is more subtle than the abdominal breath. Bring your awareness to the outside edges of your ribcage with each breath. See if you can feel the ribs expanding as you take five breaths with this thoracic focus.
- ✓ Finally, bring your finger tips to your collar bones so the elbows are outstretched and the whole lung area is expansive.
- ✓ You may well be imagining rather than feeling at this point but aim to get a sense of each breath filling the very back of the lungs. Keep your focus here for five breaths.

How did that feel?

4/2 – Mind, body, heart and soul

Psychosynthesis is an unusual psychological approach in that it's very holistic. When you think of your own life and general approach to things, are you more:

   i. cognitive ('mind'), thinking everything through?
   ii. emotional (I'll say 'heart'), going with how you feel about things?
   iii. embodied ('body'), having real somatic awareness?
   iv. transpersonal (some say 'soul' but you don't have to believe in that to think of something beyond the person) or spiritual?

In an ideal world, while we all have our preferences, we synthesise, come together, and become better able to integrate *all* aspects of ourselves.

What might you do today to boost your awareness of one of the less familiar ways of navigating your world? For most of us, becoming more embodied is a challenge. Whether we're emotional, more cognitive or even spiritual, stopping to observe physical sensations **(6/2 and 14/8)** or even just noticing the breath **(7/1)** can be a great start. Go easy on yourself and have fun experimenting.

5/2 – Mindful Minute

Conscious breathing has so many benefits. It brings us straight into the present moment and into our bodies. Mindful or conscious breathing strengthens the prefrontal cortex. This part of the brain helps us make good decisions, relate well to people, calm the more primitive parts of the brain down and concentrate.

We don't have to overwhelm ourselves – we've been breathing just fine our whole lives. And we're still alive to prove it. **7/1, 8/1** and **9/1** go into more detail but today, as you allow your breath to slow and begin to feel relaxed, time yourself.

For 30 seconds, count your natural, calm breaths (one inhalation plus exhalation equals one breath). Double it for the number of breaths you take in one minute.

Five to six for an adult under six feet tall is ideal but lots of people breathe much faster. As we practice, our breath naturally slows so be honest with yourself. Your number is a tool to enable you to take a minute, whenever you get the chance, without needing a stopwatch.

I learned this from Liz Hall, author of *Mindful Coaching*. It's a great way to remind ourselves that while there are all sorts of benefits to longer meditations **(1/1)**, we *can* change our bodies and our minds, simply by pausing for a minute and counting however many complete breaths are in our Mindful Minute.

6/2 – Track your charge

Any time we blush, shake, feel nauseous, get turned on, or feel *any* kind of sensation – whether we label it good or bad - we have a reaction. Anodea Judith, author of *Chakra Yoga, Eastern Body, Western Mind* (and more – www.sacredcentres.com), calls this perfectly natural life force (prana, chi, whatever you want to call it) 'charge'. Like electricity. Neither good nor bad.

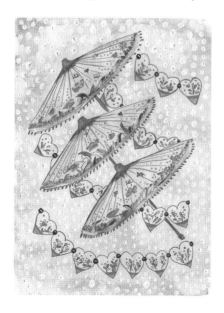

By spending less time judging ourselves for feeling however we're feeling and instead tuning *into* the charge (sensation or feeling), we can take whatever life throws at us and *harvest* that charge. A lot of my work over the past 15 plus years has been about *releasing* said charges, from anxiety, trauma, stress or other issues so this is one of my favourite of the 366 ideas for self-care.

Notice how you feel right now. Any areas of tension? Heat? Cold? Tingling, tightness, openness, anything at all? Where do you feel it? Say, 'Hello, life force! What'cha doing?' or whatever words help *you* to befriend it and be curious rather than judging and potentially repressing it. What does it *want* to do? What's blocking it? How might you harvest it?

7/2 – Coherent breathing

Dr Patricia Gerbarg, one of the guest lecturers when I did my initial yoga therapy training, introduced me to the concept of coherent breathing. It has been used to reduce post-traumatic stress (PTS) symptoms, anxiety, insomnia, aggression, depression, fatigue, impulsivity and inattention. There are no contraindications.

While Stephen Elliot named it coherent breathing, Paul Lehrer called it resonant breathing. Zen Buddhist monks use it during deep meditation and it's also taught in Qi Gong. It can be done with Ujjayi **(6/4)** or without and promotes cardiorespiratory resonance and sympathovagal balance **(29/2)**.

Best of all, it's really simple. Aim to slow the breath to five or six complete breaths per minute. Each inhalation and exhalation is approximately six seconds. This is different to our Mindful Minutes **(5/2)** as here we are actively slowing the breath down. There, we were noticing our natural relaxed breath rate.

*You can buy Dr Gerbarg and her colleagues' **Respire 1** CD, which paces five breaths per minute with sound cues, from www.coherence.com*

8/2 – What tone of voice do you use when you talk to yourself?

I recently blogged about how years of therapy and doing this work hadn't embedded a kind inner voice as my default (as opposed to when consciously coaching myself) in the same way that adopting a rescue cat did.

From the time I brought Rainbow MagnifiCat home, my intention was to keep her in parasympathetic (rest/digest **(9/1)**) mode as much as possible, apart from when playing, which is lifting, activating sympathetic mode, but in a friendly way. The world is stimulating enough and her feline friends are sometimes more like frenemies.

By talking to her as gently and soothingly as possible, even first thing in the morning, when she's knocked something over or when I wake up in the night, I've naturally become more soothing in my own self talk, even sometimes calling myself 'Kitten'.

I'm not at all suggesting we pressure ourselves to become paragons of calm and patience 24/7 but it's been a wonderful practice for me that you may want to experiment with.

Maybe you've noticed similar with your dog, goat, hamster or baby?

9/2 – Opening our hearts

With Valentine's Day approaching, we're looking at some more heart openers.

We can do this emotionally and mentally with Metta meditations **(15/2)**. We can also do this physically, by expanding our heart area, physically opening up to love, connection and all the good life has to offer.

When our posture allows our hearts to be open, we're more likely to connect and listen and love. As with all of these tips, they're for you to play with. Some days, it may feel like the most natural thing in the world to open up, physically, emotionally, mentally and even spiritually. Other days, you may feel too vulnerable. While vulnerability, as Brené Brown's research shows **(27/6)**, is a key ingredient for wholehearted living, we don't have to force anything.

Notice the times it's easier and you feel strong and open hearted. And notice the times when you want to allow your heart to take a duvet day. Be open-hearted and compassionate with yourself instead of forcing anything.

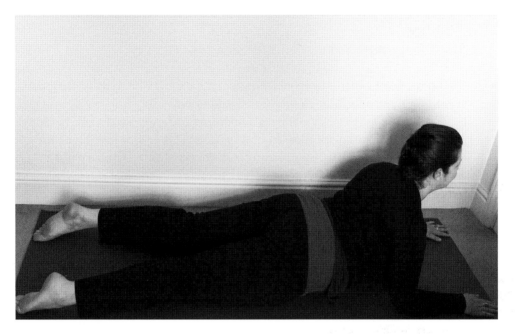

10/2 – Sphinx

This is one of my favourite heart openers **(9/2)**. Much of the body remains grounded so the heart can open in a protected, safe way.

- ✓ If you want to try it, start by lying on your belly with your head, neck and spine aligned. You can release any heart aches and blocks through the heart centre, into the earth, knowing they can be recycled, energetically, for the benefit of the planet.
- ✓ Move the elbows so they are under the shoulders. Lift the heart centre and eyes so you're looking ahead. Drop the shoulder blades and notice your breath. Hold for five breaths if that feels good.

As well as helping us lift our mood, Sphinx strengthens the spine and abdominal muscles. It's a gentle backbend so we can really tune into the level that's right for us at any given time.

Similarly, when it comes to opening our hearts off the yoga mat, we can become attuned to the degree of intensity we choose at any time.

11/2 – Restorative Fish

This time, our hearts can expand even more, facing the heavens while the whole body remains fully grounded and supported.

Using a yoga bolster or cushions and pillows, start by sitting with your legs in front of you and bolster lengthways behind you. It may be touching your lower back or a fist distance away. Allow your torso to release onto the bolster at a degree that feels good. If it's uncomfortable to lie back directly onto the bolster, you may want a folded blanket on top of it to make the backbend less intense.

It should feel delicious and restorative, no effort – we're all different and if your body doesn't like it, experiment with different heights (maybe putting a blanket on the bolster) or don't do it. As always, you know what's best for you. You can use blankets to cover you, too if you're cold or feeling vulnerable while still wanting to play with it. Sometimes, Restorative Fish feels amazing, other times, maybe vulnerable.

Relax there for five minutes. Stay longer if you have time and are enjoying it or shorter if that's all you can squeeze in. Allow yourself to come out of it slowly. It's a deeper backbend than it feels when resting in it so put your weight on your elbows to gently ease out of it.

This back bend can help lift the mood and open the lungs and shoulders as well as our hearts. Restorative Fish can also be interesting for a Metta (loving kindness) meditation **(15/2)** from here. It enables us to send that loving kindness from a supported and expanded heart centre.

It allows us to ponder all the good life has to offer and literally open our hearts to it all.

12/2 – Drama triangle

Dr Stephen B Karpman made this dynamic famous and it's a great quick question to ponder.

Are we in Victim, Rescuer or Perpetrator mode?

Which is our default setting? Do things keep happening to us? Do we forget that *we* might be the common denominator? That even when much is out of our control there's always *something* we can do to get out of that seductive Victim position? **(16/1)**

Maybe we're more comfortable as a Rescuer **(14/1)**. Even if no one *needs* rescuing, there we are, ready and willing to help. Getting trapped in this role can be exhausting as we try fixing the world. We can also be really irritating. By taking on this role unconsciously, we might even be contributing to keeping someone feeling helpless and unable to rescue themselves.

And then there's the Perpetrator. Often, the hardest for us to identify with. Oh no, we'd *never* behave like that. And yet, being human, we all have the capacity for everything. Denying our inner perpetrators means they can get repressed and come out in shadow.

Even the sweetest, kindest seeming Rescuer or Victim might be seen by *someone* as a Perpetrator. As you think about your romantic and other relationships, ask yourself how you might step out of your default role and enjoy more freedom.

13/2 – What would you say and to whom if you weren't afraid of rejection?

One of the great things about having an open heart and living wholeheartedly, is that it's a powerful way to be present. Amy Cuddy's work **(26/11)** in this area shows that expansive poses are almost all open hearted poses. This supports Brené Brown's work around shame and vulnerability **(27/6)** and how there's strength in vulnerability which can lead to wholehearted living.

Not that it's easy. As with everything, it's a practice. Today, you might ask yourself what you would like to say to someone (the first person who springs to mind. You don't have to *do* it, just imagine it and decide for yourself) if you weren't afraid of rejection. It might be someone you'd like to get to know better. It might be a partner of decades. It might be a friend whose actions have hurt you.

Imagine yourself expressing yourself, with compassion for yourself and them, from a wholehearted place. How does that feel?

14/2 – Happy Valentine's Day!

Whether you're single or loved up, you might want to detach yourself a little (just for a moment) from the commercial drama of Valentine's Day. Pay attention to how you're feeling. Is anything frustrating you about your current situation? Not being able to script someone else's gifts/declarations of love/responses like a Shonda Rhimes show*? Are you feeling pressure to be romantic when you don't feel like it or you're cut off from it all?

Feel your feelings. Just for a few moments. What do they tell you about what you need and want? How can you take steps to meet these needs?

A more loving and compassionate attitude to ourselves can help us improve *all* of our relationships. Picking one of them (whether romantic or not), how might you be more loving and accepting with *that one person*? Is this easier or more challenging to imagine than accepting yourself?

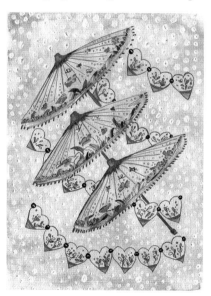

15/2 – Metta meditations

I start every morning with Metta/Loving Kindness. I learned a trauma-sensitive form during my initial yoga therapy training and appreciate its heart expanding qualities. In 2008, research published in the *Journal of*

---

* *Grey's Anatomy, Scandal, Private Practice, The Catch* and more.

Personality and Social Psychology showed that the positive emotions Metta builds help us feel more purpose **(7/12)** and satisfaction in life as well as reducing symptoms of illness.

Be gentle with yourself. Just as some days we're more physically flexible and strong or have better concentration, our compassion can shift. If we're having a tough time, it may be challenging.

Start with yourself and say:

> 'May I be happy and healthy, peaceful and at ease.'
> 'May I be able to take care of myself joyfully.'
> 'May I possess the courage, wisdom, patience and determination to manage life's challenges.'

Pause and let each sentence resonate.

Then you send it out – to a loved one, to someone you may find challenging (or if you don't feel up to that in the moment, another loved one), maybe the people in your town, continent … the individual steps are limitless. It just starts and finishes with you.

I include the day's (and past, present and future) clients and students, my neighbourhood, loved ones, other groups or individuals around the globe. These can include groups I want to do more to help but often feel helpless about, like refugees, people affected by a natural disaster, the rest of the UK and Europe and so on.

Once you've done a few rounds, do one for everyone on the planet (again, notice any resistance and be kind to yourself) and come back to yourself. Pause and notice the effects.

The HeartMath Institute has researched the electromagnetic field of the heart and while I've not been wired up doing Metta personally, I can definitely sense the expansion and healing.

It also beats tears when concerned about people I can't actually do anything about. I often send Metta to people I see on the street or well up about seeing the news. We can be creative with it. It can be especially lovely to practice in an expansive position such as Restorative Fish **(11/2)**.

16/2 – Nonviolent Communication

Developed by Marshall Rosenberg and used around the globe in areas of conflict as well as in homes and in our own heads, Nonviolent Communication (NVC) helps us communicate from the heart.

This doesn't mean it's easy. Asking for what we need and want and being able to hear what others need and want can be tough.

'The clearer we are about what we want back, the more likely we are to get it,' writes Rosenberg in *Nonviolent Communication – A Language of Life.*

He encourages us to use anger as a wakeup call, to help us get clearer about what we need.

17/2 – Giraffes and Jackals

NVC is all about empathy. Giraffes and Jackals are tools Rosenberg uses as a quick, simple reminder.

Giraffes, having the largest heart of any land mammal, are what we're aiming for. To sense and express our own feelings and needs (Giraffe In) and sensing, feeling and listening to others' feelings and needs (Giraffe Out). Giraffes represent compassionate communication.

Being human, we often take the Jackal approach. This is blaming, judging and attacking ourselves for whatever we feel or need (Jackal In). Blaming and attacking others for their feelings and needs (Jackal Out) is also unhelpful.

I feel badly for the maligned jackals but Rosenberg had to pick an animal to represent these unhelpful communication styles. I wish they had some good PR. Still, wondering 'Giraffe or Jackal?' is another tool to aid mindfulness around our self-talk and the way we communicate with others.

Pausing periodically, we can ask ourselves if we notice any Jackal (In or Out) tendencies. Honouring the times we're coming from a more Giraffe (In or Out) space can create enormous shifts in our relationships with others and for our own peace of mind.

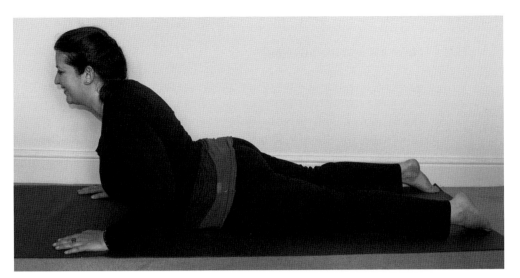

18/2 – Mini Cobra

Mini Cobra's benefits include strengthening the arms, helping us with better boundaries and integrating rest and growth. It builds wrist and arm strength, aids adrenal and kidney function and, of course, opens the heart from a grounded place.

Contraindications include headaches, lower back issues, pregnancy, bipolar and some post-traumatic stress symptoms.

A small study published in *Human Physiology* (2004) found higher testosterone and lower cortisol in blood serum of participants after holding Cobra for three minutes. This research helped inspire Amy Cuddy **(26/11)** to look at expansive poses for people not necessarily wanting to do yoga.

- ✓ Lying on your belly with your head, neck and spine nicely aligned, place your hands under your shoulders with the fingers spread out. Lengthen the legs and ground the toes, thighs and front of the pelvis.
- ✓ Keeping the pubic bone on the ground, slowly lift the head and heart centre up, keeping the elbows close to the sides and pressing through the hands.
- ✓ Feel that smooth curved extension through the cervical spine and gaze in front. Slide the shoulders down and notice what's happening with the breath. Are you able to keep it controlled?
- ✓ Aim to hold it (you're probably very aware of your upper arms) for five full breaths if that feels good then come back down to rest on your belly.

19/2 – 'I love life and life loves me'

While this sounds very like Louise Hay, it was an affirmation on the Sun card in an Aleister Crowley Tarot deck I had when I was younger. After my morning meditation, I fling my arms out wide and say it aloud.

Some mornings, I believe it. Other times, it feels a little vulnerability-inducing so I know to be extra gentle and patient with myself.

How do you feel when you express your love for life? Do you believe life loves you back?

When you finish, you can hug yourself and, if you want, repeat the hug on the other side for balance.

20/2 – Keeping the heart open in Warrior II pose

Warrior II is a great pose for building confidence and enhancing our capacity to draw on our inner warriors. While using up stress hormones, we also become more able to stay present with whatever's happening. If we have a tendency to give up too easily, holding Warrior II pose and gradually building up can help us transfer that warrior strength to our lives off the mat. If our tendency is to endure too much, we can challenge ourselves (especially in a class) by paying extra attention to our own needs. Maybe coming out of the pose earlier if that's what's right for us. While Warrior II benefits all the chakras, it's especially good for the base **(9/7)**, solar plexus **(11/7)** and heart chakras **(25/1 and 12/7)**. And it fits with Amy Cuddy's Power Pose criteria **(26/11)**.

- ✓ Stand towards the front of your yoga mat, with your feet hip distance apart and your hips square to the short edge of the mat.
- ✓ Take the left foot back to a comfortable distance having the heel parallel with the front (right) foot. Use the long, straight edge of your mat as a guideline.
- ✓ Bend the right knee and ensure you can see the tips of the toes over the knee so you're not putting excess pressure on the ankle. It activates the thigh muscles so is a great preparation for Wheel **(15/11)**.

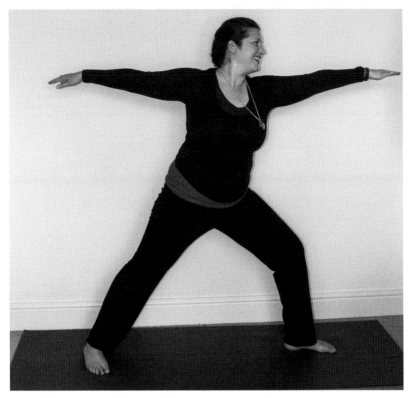

- ✓ Raise the arms so they're parallel to the floor and create a straight line. Keep the torso upright and heart centre open. Imagine your inner warrior having all the spiritual, emotional and physical power required for any situation you may be facing off the yoga mat. Remember, an open heart helps us stand strong and compassionate.
- ✓ Maintain the central axis with the pelvis, heart and head vertically aligned.
- ✓ Control the breath and aim to hold (for Power Pose benefits) for at least one minute on each side.

21/2 – Bow pose

Bow helps us use up stress hormones. It's also grounding and tones the back,

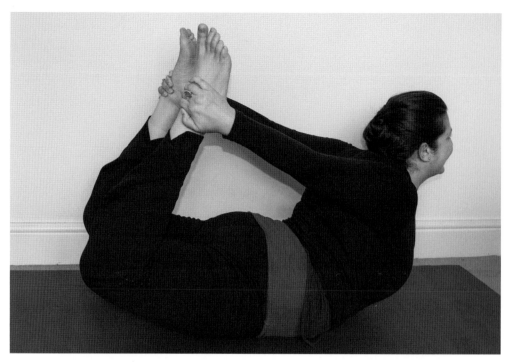

buttocks and legs. Uplifting and energising while in Bow, in the longer term, the pose helps us build greater autonomic control: Controlling our breath in such poses means that, with practice, we become better at handling bigger physical and emotional stresses without the old impact.

Bow is also helpful for women with hormone imbalances. It can ease symptoms associated with menopause, menstruation and postnatal depression. Like all backbends, Bow can help us lift our mood.

- ✓ Start by lying on your belly. Bend your knees, keeping them in line with the hips and shoulders and take both hands to both ankles. If you're unable to reach on both sides, do Half Bow (first stretching one side then the other) rather than being off balance.
- ✓ Grounding the pelvis, rock back with both hands and hold the outer feet or ankles. Keep drawing the shoulders away from the ears and lengthen the neck. Push the feet into the hands to lift more.
- ✓ Notice the breath and aim for as much control as possible, breathing into the belly and lower lungs, aiming for that longer exhalation **(9/1)**.
- ✓ If it feels OK for your neck, look forwards or up.

✓ To come out of Bow, gently release the ankles or feet and come back onto the belly, resting face down for a few complete breaths to allow the system to come back down again. Lifting and lowering the system with rest poses after dynamic ones helps us retrain the autonomic nervous system **(9/1)**.

22/2 – Up Dog

Part of many Sun Salutation sequences, Upward Facing Dog or Up Dog helps strengthen the spine, arms, wrists, shoulders, chest, lungs and abdomen. Incredibly heart opening, it can also strengthen the internal organs, including increasing lung capacity. It can lift our mood as well as energising us.

✓ Lying on your belly, come up onto the palms of the hands (which should be below the elbows and shoulders to avoid any pressure for the lower back), extending the arms and lengthening the neck as much as is comfortable.

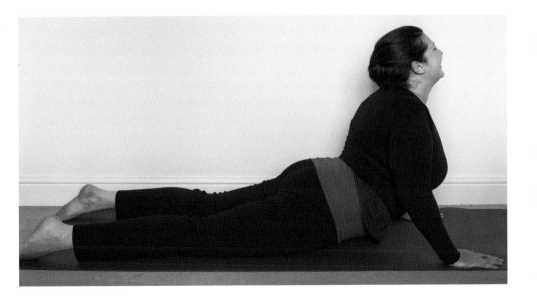

- ✓ Ideally, just the tips of the toes and palms of the hands touch the mat as you open into Up Dog.
- ✓ During Sun Salutations, come from Up Dog into Down Dog **(30/4)** or, if practicing it on its own, come back to rest on your belly. Notice the breath and how you feel during and afterwards.

23/2 – Kapalabhati

This cleansing breath helps us expel stagnant prana (energy). It tones the diaphragm, respiratory tract and muscles of the abdominal cavity. When practiced between Ujjayi **(6/4)**, it helps retrain the autonomic nervous system **(9/1)**.

Kapalabhati can also lower heart rate and blood pressure (after calming Ujjayi breath afterwards), boost vagal tone **(29/2)** and is great for respiratory or weight issues. Keep tissues nearby – you may need them.

Be careful if you have any problems with blood pressure and avoid when pregnant or if you feel anxious about it. Although it calms the system overall, it's a lifting breath while doing it.

- ✓ If it's comfortable, kneel (if not, sit) with a straight spine and exhale, forcefully through your nostrils. Unusually for pranayama (breath practices), this is all about the exhalation. The inhalation happens naturally here. While you can focus on the abdomen pushing out with each forced exhalation, I've found it easier since Emma Turnbull **(3/5)** suggested imagining a pea shooting out of my nose.
- ✓ To begin, play with ten forced exhales per round then take one slow exhale as you bow towards the ground before starting a second round. Repeat a third time.

With practice, you'll get faster but start slow and easy and do it at a pace that suits you now.

24/2 – What would you do if you cared about yourself?

Sometimes, the leap from self-loathing or simply bleugh to self-love can feel too risky. On these days - or months or moments - we can simply ask ourselves, 'What would I do if I cared about myself?'

We can ask ourselves this simple question before making any decision, from accepting (or extending) an invitation to before eating, deciding whether to exercise or taking the next baby step along the path to a long held dream.

How does it feel to tune into that part of yourself that *knows* the most caring choice in any given moment?

25/2 – Tune into your inner guidance

What do you call that whole, wisest, most loving and compassionate part of yourself? In psychosynthesis, it's known as the Self. The part of us that observes all the other parts with curiosity **(7/6)** and compassion. Other traditions have other names for it.

Tara Mohr, author of *Playing Big*, calls it the Inner Mentor. Art Giser **(3/1)** says Miraculous Self. Gabrielle Bernstein calls this inner guide the ING. Sonia Choquette, Spirit or Sixth Sense and others, the soul.

What happens when we pause for a moment and tune into what this part of us wants us to do next?

Learning to listen and act on this inner wisdom – which we can access anytime anywhere – can be transformative. As with everything, it's a practice. When is it easiest? How might you do more of the things that help you honour this wisdom?

26/2 – Other people's emergencies

Years ago, a yoga therapy friend, Lou Kitchener (www.yogahappy.co.uk) made me laugh about a stressful situation by quoting her lovely dad: 'Poor planning on your part does not constitute an emergency on my part.'

I never met him but, over the years, imagining him calmly saying these words has helped me pause and avoid getting sucked into all sorts of sticky situations. I've never actually said the words aloud in such a situation, but often, just imagining doing so makes me smile and release that sense of pressure that has nothing to do with me.

I wanted to honour him here and share his advice as it can make us laugh - but only inwardly. I'm not suggesting we laugh openly at those who may already be beating themselves up for such poor planning - at others' urgent demands. It can take some of the heat out of unrealistic expectations.

27/2 – Modelling imperfection

Another yoga therapy friend, Maya, had a big impact on me, years ago, when she made a mistake. Instead of shame spiralling as I was prone to do, she simply shrugged, smiled and said, 'Modelling imperfection.' I've repeated it countless times with students, clients and myself. It creates freedom and connection rather than shame.

As my old Improvisation teacher, Steve Roe **(26/6)**, used to say, as long as we're not surgeons, mistakes are brilliant. The training I did with him, while not directly related to my work, really helped me relax into what I do.

When you catch yourself being human, how does it feel to say, 'Just modelling imperfection?' with a shrug?

We can recover and correct far faster by smiling at ourselves and moving on.

28/2 - A different kind of cycling

Sick of feeling invincible one day then, the next, like each breath is wasting oxygen someone else could benefit from? Lisa Lister's *Code Red* (SHE Press, 2015) helps us get to know our menstrual cycles so we can plan to do different kinds of things (and make time for extra self-care) throughout. We can boost our productivity, effectiveness, joy and sense of ease by honouring each phase.

As the moon has its phases and year has its seasons, we women have our own cycles. **6/3, 25/6, 29/9** and **18/12** give for more information about typical phases and learning to appreciate every day of the month.

If you're a man, this may still be of interest as you can become better attuned to the women in your life.

Find out more about Lisa Lister (including her latest book,* Love Your Lady Landscape *(Hay House, 2016) at www.thesassyshe.com

29/2 – The vagus

80 per cent of the signals between body and brain go from the body to the brain. They are carried up via this 10th cranial nerve, the vagus. When we remember this, it's easier to motivate ourselves to change the way we're breathing, sitting, standing or moving in order to improve the way we feel. Having used our body and breath to change the way we feel, the brain can send stronger 'All is well' calming signals to the whole body. This is more effective than forcing ourselves to calm down by mentally yelling, 'Relax!' at ourselves.

Certain breath practices **(7/1)**, chanting **(22/1)** and yoga poses as well as exercise in general all boost vagal tone, helping us better handle life's ups and downs.

March

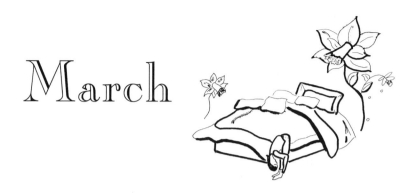

This month's tips include space clearing, natural rhythms, becoming detectives into our sleep patterns, mindfulness of the breath, body and thoughts and more yoga.

1/3 – What's your dragon tail like?

Hapus Dydd Dewi Sant! (Happy St David's Day!) I learned today's tool from somatic coach-therapist, Clare Myatt (www.claremyatt.co.uk). She credits the Strozzi Institute (www.strozziinstitute.com) as inspiration and originators.

Having grounded and centred yourself **(13/3)**, imagine a line of energy going down your spine from the nape of your neck to your tailbone.

Imagine it continuing on, growing into a dragon's tail. This tail is filled with the energy of all the people who've ever loved you, all your achievements, skills experience and all you've survived. How does yours look and feel?

Mine (weirdly) makes me dance a little. Since I've been working with it, it's gone from a scaly but feminine dragon tail to plush but very strong red velvet. I no longer worry about it getting dirty or damaged.

Trust your own inner wisdom regarding whatever emerges for you. Our tails give us gravitas. They change the way we walk. Similar to Art Giser's magnet clearing **(3/1)**, they remind us the world is a safe, welcoming place.

2/3 – Singing

Like chanting **(22/1)**, singing is brilliant for naturally elongating the exhalation **(9/1)** and helping us find our voices. If you drive, belting out your favourites in your own little bubble can be a great way to use your voice, not just for that tune but to help you tune into what you want to express in your life.

When we sing with others, we can even boost our oxytocin levels **(7/11)**. Whether you stick to singing in your car or shower, regularly wow at Karaoke or even perform professionally, notice the times your voice feels strong and true.

And notice the times you feel more shy. Play with different styles of music and tunes and have fun with finding your voice.

3/3 – Dressing

Do you feel like you wear the same thing day after day? That you are stuck in a rut?

Years ago, Angela Buttolph presented a delightful TV show called *My Week of Dressing Dangerously*. People would hand over control of their wardrobes for a week. They'd go to work and out on dates wearing crazy costumes chosen by Angela to bring out hidden aspects of their personalities. We don't have to go to such extremes but can pause to imagine the woman or man we'd like to be.

How would you be if you dressed differently? I'm not suggesting you get into debt or anything, but how might you experiment with different styles? When you think about different subpersonalities **(10/1)**, how might *they* dress?

Is there anything you're ready to release from your wardrobe?

Anything you wish you were to be brave enough to wear?

Use your clothes and makeup, if you wear it, to express yourself. Experiment. Have fun.

4/3 – Lion pose

I'm never sure how new students will react to Lion pose but I continue encouraging them to roar. Even if they don't do it in class, learning it might encourage them to play with it at home. Benefits include boosting circulation in the tongue and throat and exercising and strengthening the face and throat muscles. The longer exhalation helps calm the nervous system **(9/1)**.

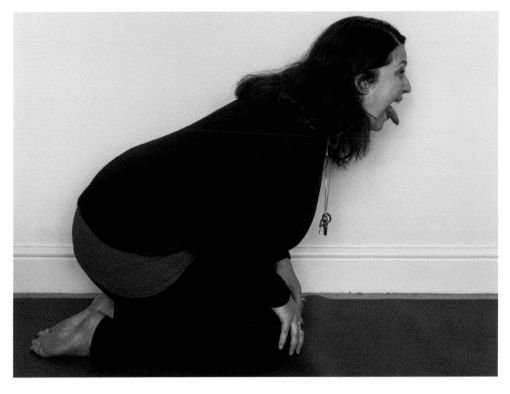

I teach it by encouraging students and clients to ponder current stressors – anything they'd like to just roar away – before moving into Lion. Even the act of honouring whatever is stressing us out in any given moment helps release some of the energy around it.

- ✓ Resting in Child **(28/10)** or similar, think of up to six stressors you'd rather not have in your life right now.
- ✓ Come into a low kneeling position, placing the hands on your knees. If this isn't comfortable, adjust.

- ✓ Widen your eyes, rolling them up as you ROAR, stretching your tongue out, make a forced 'Ahhhh' sound. It actually sounds more like I imagine a snake would sound than a lion.
- ✓ Fold forwards and then come back up to the original position. Repeat a couple of times, each time, roaring away a different stress.
- ✓ Repeat another three times or move into Crazy Lion. As you fold forward, move your head and neck and torso in all sorts of directions as you let yourself go. When you complete your six rounds, come back to your kneeling (or other starting) position and notice how you feel.

It's entirely possible that the beaming faces I often see as we complete Lion in classes are at least partially down to relief at having *done* it but it's great fun so do feel free to play with it, if you want to.

5/3 – Spring cleaning, space clearing

In the past, stronger daylight showed up dirt from fireplaces and winter in general. Fortunately, cleaning is a less arduous task for us now. We can take advantage of the urge to clean and clear by visualising as we vacuum, imagining releasing any and all stagnant, old, unnecessary energies as we clean. Ridding the home, office, car etc. and ourselves of any blocks. Opening windows lets fresh air blast away old beliefs that may be holding us back. Be creative and have fun with it.

Nature abhors a vacuum so think about what you're making space for. Play with some ENLP space clearing and setting **(2/1)** to bring more of the good stuff into your home and life. While you may never *love* vacuuming, it can at least feel extra beneficial.

6/3 – Pre-ovulation

Many women find this spring-like, waxing (growing) lunaresque part of our cycle great for understanding, memory and logic. Our creativity **(6/6)** can be heightened and we often have the stamina and drive to make our dreams a reality. It's a great time to put ourselves out there as we feel more extraverted and often want to be seen and heard. Increased oestrogen levels also make us more tolerant of our loved ones and strangers.

Lisa Lister **(28/2)** suggests setting intentions, enjoying being a beginner and protecting new ideas and ourselves.

7/3 – Sleep detective

There are many remedies for insomnia but we're all different. Rather than psyching yourself out thinking you can never give up your bedtime screen time, even though you know it inhibits melatonin production, become a detective into your own sleep habits.

Play with all the tips you want to and rate them according to how helpful they are for you. Then you'll have a clearer idea of how to create a soothing bedtime ritual for yourself. It may feel dull – it may even bore you to sleep! - but logging what supports and hinders a good night's sleep will help you make tweaks. This can help you transform your relationship to bedtime (and wake up more energised).

What routines help you get a better night's sleep?

8/3 – Self soothing talk when wide awake

The last thing we want to do when wide awake in the early hours is probably the most natural thing *to* do: stress about *exactly* how exhausted we're going to be tomorrow. We calculate the swiftly diminishing hours or minutes of sleep before the dreaded alarm. But these thoughts trigger the stress response **(3/4)**, making sleep practically impossible physiologically. To sleep, we need to be in rest/digest mode, activating the parasympathetic branch of the autonomic nervous system **(9/1)**.

Even when we feel like the biggest liar since Pinocchio, we can tell ourselves that we're going to be absolutely fine tomorrow. Even if we only get five minutes' sleep.

The breath **(7/1)** can help us calm our system. If that doesn't help, a body scan **(4/4)**, yoga nidra **(9/3)** or a little yoga might. We can support ourselves in entering the Relaxation Response **(1/1)**.

9/3 – Yoga Nidra

This translates as yogic sleep and helps us enter such a deep state of relaxation, we go through several different states of brain wave activity. It increases dopamine release, a feel good, motivational hormone **(16/12)**, by 65 per cent, according to research published in *Cognitive Brain Research* (T.W. Kjaer et al, 2002). It can even support us in creating new neural pathways, making healthier behaviours and beliefs much easier. A sankalpa – positive intention, resolve or affirmation – is something we allow to come from the heart. Repeating the same one over time (to allow those new neural pathways to develop) at the start and finish provide even more benefits from this relaxing practice.

Ideally, we stay awake (we're aiming to harness that state between sleep and wakefulness) throughout. We stay as still as possible but it's a relaxation practice so if we need to move or snooze, we can honour our own body's wisdom.

Yoga Nidra not only helps with stress, anxiety, post-traumatic stress and helps lower high blood pressure but can ease symptoms of migraines, heart disease, diabetes, cancer and asthma.

10/3 – Pendulums – First Aid with crystals

This is so simple and effective, yet every time I do it, I'm astonished at how magical it feels.

- ✓ Choose, cleanse and dedicate **(25/8)** your crystal pendulum and then hold it over an area of the body that feels fine. Notice the direction it swings in and make a note of it. Hold it over another healthy area and note that. And a third.
- ✓ Now hold it over an area that feels painful. Is it moving in the opposite direction? Even though you're absolutely not making it do that?
- ✓ Swing it manually in the direction you've calibrated as healthy for your body right now and keep swinging it that way for a few moments.
- ✓ When you feel you've done enough, test it by holding the pendulum and noticing how it's moving on its own. Sometimes, it may still move in the unhealthy direction or it may be more jerky as if it's changing course.
- ✓ Go back to manually swinging in the healthy way and keep testing until it naturally moves, without your help,

Obviously, use the advantages of modern medicine too and see a doctor if necessary. Crystals **(22/8)** can be wonderful but they're complementary not alternative. Please be sensible.

11/3 – Bridge pose

- ✓ Lie on your back with head, neck and spine aligned, arms alongside the body, palms down. Draw the feet towards the torso with bent knees over the ankles. Gently inhale rising up and exhale back down.
- ✓ After a few breaths like this, you may want to hold the pose, lifting

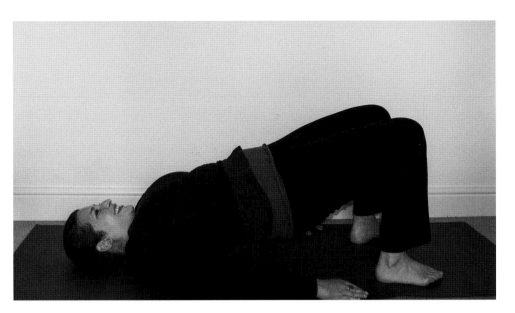

the hips towards the heavens, opening the heart centre and noticing the breath. Don't have the feet so close to the torso that the hips jut forward.

✓ Keep the inner thighs active (maybe using a block between the knees) and when you've taken a few (five if that feels good) complete breaths, gently come back down to the ground and stretch in whatever way feels best for you.

It's a balancing pose, both grounding and energising. The heart is open and it helps build power and lung capacity as well as relieving lower back tension. Holding it for a short time (or simply inhaling lifting up and exhaling down) can be helpful for high blood pressure.

It also helps us ponder gaps between where we were and where we want to be. We can reflect on what we've already bridged in our lives, knowing we can do the same with current obstacles.

12/3 – More on Metta

Traditionally, after ourselves and someone we love **(15/2)**, we move to someone more neutral and then onto someone we find challenging. Sometimes, sending loving kindness to ourselves is challenging enough, so be kind to yourself as you build up to this.

Some days, our heart centres feel strong and balanced and we can send genuine Metta to people we're really struggling with. Other times, the attempt could be counterproductive. Similarly, when we're feeling that much more resilient, we can send loving kindness to more challenging people, maybe to an individual, a politician or a group of people. How does that feel today?

13/3 – Grounding and centring

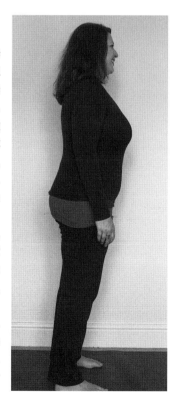

- ✓ Unlike many grounding tools, this is done with open eyes so can, especially with practice, be incredibly useful for those moments when we need to ground the most. Clare Myatt (**1/3**) recommends standing with your feet hip distance apart, both feet facing forward. Press into the soles a little, adjusting until you feel evenly balanced. Notice if your knees are locked and drop the kneecaps to release that tension.
- ✓ Notice your pelvis, belly and buttocks, releasing any tension there. Drop your shoulder blades and release any tension in your jaw. Soften your gaze and just notice, head to foot, how this feels.
- ✓ Lengthening through the spine, stand tall and straight, as if being lifted from the crown of the head, feeling your dignity. Imagine tea leaves or whatever emerges for

you, dropping and settling in your abdomen. Widen for social standing, maybe moving the hands slightly away.

✓ Then deepen, imagining a line going from in front of your lower abdomen through and behind, for gravitas. Notice how this feels. Adjust as needed. You may also want to add your Dragon's Tail **(1/3)**.

14/3 – Yogic caffeine

I learned about the concept of 'yogic caffeine' from insomnia and better-sleep specialist Lisa Sanfilippo (www.lisayogalondon.com). The mid-afternoon slump we all deal with - and often try to override with chocolate and/or coffee - can be alleviated with some yoga.

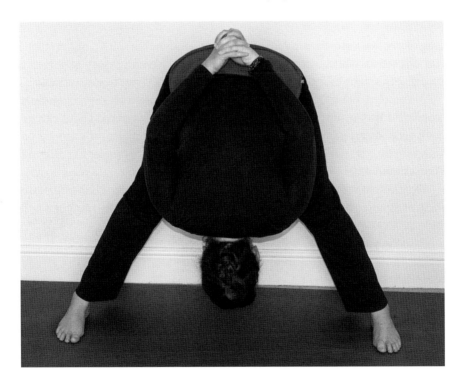

'One stretch is a Wide Legged Forward Bend,' **(18/3)** says Lisa. 'You can bend your knees if you need to - this stretches the spinal nerves and spinal muscles and brings blood flow and circulation into the upper front of the lungs, creating a stimulating effect. Let your head drop down and bring circulation into your face, creating the bio-feedback from the surge into the facial muscles that wakes you up. Bend your knees and sit on the floor.

'The next posture is called the Little Bridge pose **(11/3)**. Place the soles of the feet to the floor with your knees pointing upwards. Rest the back of your skull on the floor and gently lift your hips up. Pull your arms together to clasp your hands behind your back and breathe deeply to stretch the ribcage and abdominal muscles. The deep backbend enables the nerves in the upper back to stimulate a wakeful feeling.'

15/3 – Mother's Day / Family Constellations

One of my favourite therapy jokes is 'If it's not one thing, it's your mother.' But of course, while mothers get the worst rap (typically, they're primary care givers so our biggest influences), ancestral influences go way back.

A Family Constellations workshop with a qualified therapist can be a wonderful way of finding freedom around entrenched issues. These can go back generations including taboos, early deaths and traumas. If a workshop isn't for you, you can use toys, pebbles, shells or pieces of paper to represent yourself and others in your family.

Experiment with their placement and notice how it feels when you place them a) tuning into how things are and b) gently and gradually moving them and pausing to see how the shifts feel.

Although you may be on your own (or at a workshop), the healing can feel phenomenal and will likely improve your family relationships as you heal some of those issues.

Does anything spring to mind as in need of healing for your family?

16/3 – Metta to different body parts

I started doing this in my small yoga classes, especially ones where students had chronic pain issues and ill health. Instead of asking them to look outside of themselves **(15/2 and 12/3)**, I encouraged starting with their Selves, moving on to different parts of their body and even psyche.

For example, 'May I' (in other words, that wise, whole, observer Self part of you **(21/8)**) 'be happy and healthy peaceful and at ease...' and so on.

Afterwards, choose a part of yourself - physical or personality (maybe subpersonality **(10/1)** or universal strength **(31/5)** trait) you love and accept.

Then, of course, a part you find more challenging. Maybe a subpersonality you struggle with or universal strength you overplay. Perhaps a physical part you've had health issues with or a part you've introjected loathing for because it doesn't look like model's parts. This list might be long and we can work with whatever comes up.

Then, when you've exhausted (for now) all these parts, sending loving kindness to each and every one, send it to your whole self and then back to your observer Self.

Notice how each round feels.

17/3 – Seated Forward Fold

Forward folds are calming for most of us. Our energy and attention goes inwards and we're able to tune into our own breath, thoughts and feelings.

- ✓ Sit with your legs outstretched in front of you, toes pointing up at the ceiling. Ponder your desired quality if using the Relaxation Response **(1/1)**.
- ✓ Raise your arms overhead and reach for the wall in front of you, maybe imagining yourself reaching for this quality.
- ✓ Let your hands rest wherever feels best. This is about relaxation, not endurance. Even if they're above the knee, you're still benefitting from this forward fold. Maybe they reach your calves or ankles or you can clasp your hands around the soles of your feet.

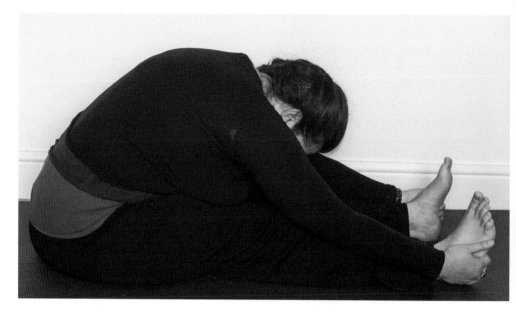

Experiment with the degree that feels best for you. You might want to hold it for five complete breaths or, if relaxing, for the three plus minutes required for the Relaxation Response.

Notice the quality of your breath. As you breathe into it, you may go more deeply into the pose or come out of it a little. Honour your own body's wisdom.

18/3 – Standing Forward Fold

This is one of my favourites but we're all built differently. If you don't find it relaxing even as you feel a pretty intense stretch, be extra kind to yourself, easing into it gently or not going down so far.

- ✓ With the feet hip distance apart and facing forward, raise your arms over your head, hinge at the hips and allow yourself to gently fold forwards to whatever degree feels good. Ensure you have at least a microbend in your knees. If it feels better to bend them more, honour that. Yoga is not a competition. Even with ourselves.

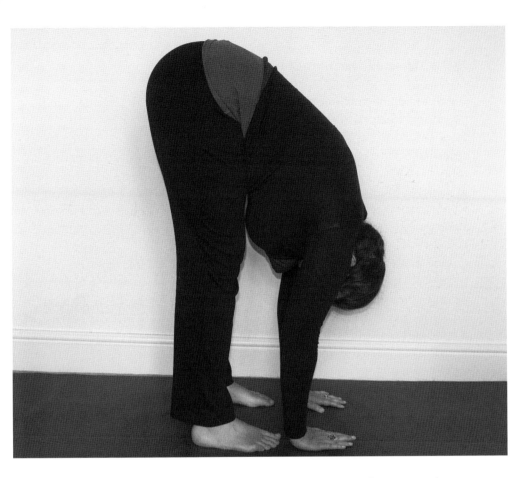

Whether your hands are under your feet, on the floor, around your ankles, on your shins or higher up, you're getting the right stretch for your body in this moment.

✓ For an extra stretch, start with the feet wide apart **(14/3)**, both facing forwards. Either bring the hands down to wherever feels best or clasp them behind the back, drawing them up as you fold forward to stretch out the shoulders.

✓ Notice your breath and aim for five complete breaths, or even three plus minutes for Relaxation Response benefits **(1/1)** if this is comfortable enough.

✓ To come up, bend the knees a little more and roll up slowly and gently. Pausing in Chair on the way up can help you avoid any light-headedness.

19/3 – National Clear Your Clutter Day

I used to be a member of the Association of Professional Declutters and Organisers when I first started coaching. I'd visit people's homes and coach them around using their environments to support themselves. While my specialisms have changed, I still want our environments to be a sanctuary for us.

I adored Marie Kondo's *Life Changing Magic of Tidying.* I followed her KonMari method over a year ago, donating dozens and dozens of bags to charity as well as binning and recycling more. Even now, she's right. No clutter.

Her 'Does it spark joy?' approach to everything alone sparks joy for me. I even declutter my Sky+ planner like this. The things we choose to keep seem to sparkle once we release stagnant energy by letting go of what no longer (or never did) serves us. Clutter clearing is also a brilliant way to ground ourselves **(13/3)** so great for base chakra **(9/7)** imbalances.

If this approach doesn't spark joy for you, there are plenty of others, like Peter Walsh (Oprah's favourite) and Life Laundry presenter Dawna Walter.

20/3 – Earth, Link, Flow meditation

This was one of the first meditations I learned, during my crystal therapy training. It remains one of my favourites.

Choosing crystals **(24/8)** to support your connection to the earth, to the divine (link) and for your flow (so this energy flows freely, helping you manifest) can be a powerful addition but you don't need them to benefit.

Start by noticing the parts of you that are in contact with the ground. Press into the floor or chair and let yourself feel that nourishing, nurturing support from the earth itself.

Notice your crown chakra **(15/7)** as you open up to divine inspiration from whatever universal energy you believe in: God/Goddess; the Universe; Your Miraculous Self **(27/3)**; that highest wisest part of yourself – whatever works for you. Allow yourself to absorb healing light from above.

Now connect with the flow energy as you allow that healing light energy from above to flow through you, releasing energies you no longer need, sending all of this into the earth so it can be recycled for the benefit of the planet.

Notice how this energy feels. When you feel ready, ground **(13/3)**, adjust your crown chakra so it's not too open for day to day life and notice the effects.

21/3 – Ostara/Spring Equinox

This is a brilliant time of year to pay special attention to balance as day and night are equal. Alternative Nostril Breathing **(7/4)**, Tree **(16/11)** and other balancing poses can also help.

Ostara is traditionally associated with helping new projects to grow. It's a gentle growth, like delicate spring bulbs. We don't want to rush things.

It's a perfect time to sort our lives out, taking stock of our personal possessions **(19/3)** and releasing what no longer serves us so the new can flourish. As well as donating or throwing away old clothes and books, we can contemplate our attitudes, habits and beliefs and release whatever we're ready to release.

Once we're free of all this, we are in a better place to take action on the projects that mean the most to us.

22/3 – World Water Day

We're lucky to have access to fresh, clean drinking water. So many people around the world don't. As well as donating to an organisation like www.wateraid.org if it feels good for you, we can take an extra moment to appreciate our own water.

Dr Emoto's life work **(2/4)** shows how powerful water is, not just as a life source but energetically. We can charge our drinking water by adding crystals, praying over it or simply sending it the qualities we'd like to absorb and be nourished by.

I use different stones for my bedside table water (for dreams and gentleness) than I do for the water I carry around with me (for fun, protection and courage). For a little aspiration and additional reminder to drink mindfully, we can add a Conscious Water flower essence water enhancer (www.consciouswater.com). Pausing beforehand, we can choose from Love, Serenity, Happiness, Rejuvenation, Sweet Dreams and Clarity, reflecting on the quality we've chosen for this mindful moment.

We can also use our bath, shower and washing up water to visualise ourselves releasing all that no longer serves and letting those energies flow, along with the dirty water, back into the earth where it can be recycled for the benefit of the planet.

23/3 – More on mindfulness of the breath

Perhaps you've been more mindful of your breathing **(7/1, 8/1** and **9/1)**, maybe practicing since early January? Notice how it feels now.

Your Mindful Minute **(5/2)** time may have changed as you've steadily worked to calm the whole system.

You may also be finding it harder to remain conscious of it as you become more practiced and it takes less concentration. Notice how your mindful breathing feels for you today. Perhaps practicing a different type of breath **(6/4** or **8/4)** can help you stay more focused on each inhalation and exhalation.

This is not about beating ourselves up. Our minds will, of course, wander but we can cultivate them, with practice. Notice your favourite breath practices and treat yourself. This is about self-care, not endurance.

24/3 – Mindfulness of the body

While we can be pretty critical of our ability to breathe mindfully **(7/1 and 23/3)**, that's *nothing* compared to the mental battering we can give our bodies as we start focusing on them. As Jon Kabat Zinn points out, mindfulness includes heartfulness. Without self-compassion, it's not as beneficial. It could even be harmful. As with so many things, it's a practice. When our thoughts are very judgmental, we can notice the parts of the body that are in contact with the ground, chair or mat. We may want to send some Metta **(16/3)** to body parts that pop into our heads with less than compassionate thoughts.

Body scans **(4/4)** and yoga nidras **(9/3)** can also help.

25/3 – Mindful thinking

It's much harder to track our thoughts than it is our breath **(7/1 and 23/3)** or even body **(24/3)** but it's worth doing. There are so many things we tell ourselves and believe without question. These might be things we worry about, limiting beliefs, and a whole host of things. The Burmese meditation technique **(13/6)** and Byron Katie's famous Work **(5/8)** can help.

But even without those, we can pause any time to pay attention to our thoughts. What kinds of things are we putting ourselves into trances by mentally repeating on autopilot? What happens when we notice our thoughts? Which thoughts feel friendlier?

Which feel familiar but awful? We can imagine them passing by, gently, easily at their own pace, maybe as if on a movie screen or as clouds in an otherwise blue sky.

Being human, our minds will wander. We can come back to mindfulness of the body and breath any time we choose. With practice, we can cultivate our minds so they become more peaceful more of the time.

26/3 – 'I feel ... I welcome ...'

My favourite mindfulness meditation comes from Buddhist Monk and peace activist, Thich Nhat Hanh.

Sitting cross legged or on a chair with your feet grounded and your spine as straight as feels comfortable, notice how you're feeling.

It may be an emotion such as 'anxious', 'stressed', 'loved up', 'livid', 'at ease', 'content' or something more physical like 'warm', 'cold', 'itchy', 'discomfort', 'pain' ... whatever the most prominent feeling is, identify it and mentally say to yourself, 'I feel [whatever it is]'.

Now (drum roll) for the sometimes tricky and other times joyful phase: 'I *welcome* [whatever the feeling is]'.

It can be quite challenging as we're typically happier welcoming certain feelings over others but even noticing which ones we're 'welcoming' through gritted teeth can be useful.

I once went from rage to gratitude in under three minutes. Not by forcing anything or trying to 'think positive' but simply by allowing and welcoming even the ickier feelings.

27/3 – Opening up to guidance

Thanks to Marianne Williamson and Gabrielle Bernstein, I finish my morning meditation each day by asking for guidance. Gabrielle suggests asking what she calls her ING (Inner Guide) but I ask my Miraculous Self, from Art Giser's ENLP **(3/1)**, 'What would you have me do? Where would you have me go? What would you have me say? And to whom?'

Susan Kennard (www.susankennard.co.uk) suggested adding, 'What do you need me to know?' and I've added other things as appropriate when working with specific issues. Opening up to that higher wisdom helps me relax into the day ahead.

28/3 – Earth hour

As we switch off the lights and the appliances we feel good about switching off for this awareness hour, we can ponder the ways technology supports and possibly hinders us. Sometimes, an hour without can feel impossible, other times, like a treat. Remember, our ancestors used to rise and sleep with the sun as not much could be done after work. We weren't built for these 24/7 lifestyles.

We can use reminders like this not just to ponder our impact on the planet but to tweak things in our own lives.

29/3 – Notice your body clock

As the clocks spring forward, we can pay some extra attention to our circadian rhythms. At what time of the day do you feel most energised? Are you begrudging the hour's sleep you've lost or are you delighted by the extra daylight?

Although we inhabit a world where 'morning people' are primed to do well at school and work, we can honour our own body clocks more than many realise, working on different types of tasks, eating and relaxing at times that best suit us. Some predict that in the future, people will look back at rigid early mornings at school as punitive for students with different body clocks. Like forcing left handed people to write with their right hands was decades earlier.

What can you do differently to honour and work *with* your natural body clock?

30/3 – Longer holds in yoga poses

A lot of interesting research is being done around yoga's therapeutic benefits. While even a short practice can be great, as we get fitter, stronger, more flexible and better able to co-ordinate the poses with the breath or control the breath, we can benefit even more. For example, holding Warrior II **(20/2)** for two minutes or longer, just one minute on each side, can bring Power Pose **(26/11)** benefits.

Holding twists for three minutes or longer aids digestion. Holding Tree **(16/11)** for up to five minutes strengthens the vestibular system.

Keep the awareness on the breath, notice how it feels in each pose and be kind to yourself, not enduring but easing into things.

31/3 – Forward folds and the Relaxation Response

Creating conditions which help us enter the Relaxation Response **(1/1, 26/1 and 8/3)** is a great way to harness the body's natural healing capacities.

If sitting or lying isn't working for you, a calming yoga pose like a Standing **(18/3)** or Seated Forward Fold **(17/3)** can be useful as the input from the muscles can help us stay more mindful and embodied. This doesn't work for everyone as some people don't find forward folds relaxing for their bodies – you know yourself best.

And, of course, our minds will still wander. It's a matter of gently bringing them back so we can gently inhale whatever quality we want more of and then exhale that same quality.

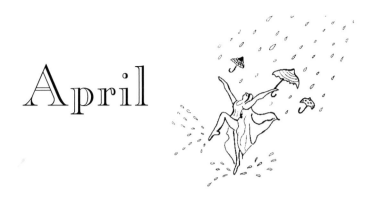

April

This month's tips include looking at how we try to fool ourselves, some of the ways in which our souls find expression in daily life, some yoga inversions and pranayama (yogic breath) practices.

1/4 – Fooling yourself?

This April Fools' Day, are you willing to be totally honest with yourself about how you fool yourself? I can laugh at myself now but for a long time, even as a health journalist writing about nutrition, I would tell myself that yum yums were *fine* for breakfast. Their deliciousness made up for any alleged lack of nutritional value and excess sugar.

Now, most days, I have more sensible breakfasts like scrambled egg on wholewheat toast or porridge, albeit with a heaped soup spoon of brown sugar, cinnamon and milk. I have more energy and it feels like I'm taking better care of myself.

What springs to mind for you? Maybe it's around food and exercise choices? Finances? Your relationships? Your style? Work? Noticing it doesn't mean you *have* to stop trying to fool yourself about whatever's not working in your life. It's entirely up to you.

2/4 – Loving every cell

Dr Emoto's **(22/3)** research around emotions affecting the chemical composition of water has been pretty revolutionary. So much of the human body is also made up of water, it's no wonder we feel things so deeply.

We can start with our own thoughts. Noticing thoughts of self-loathing and hate is a start. I'm not suggesting we leap from that to self-love but that we at least *start* curbing that hate speech in our thoughts.

Body scans **(4/4)** can help with this and you might also enjoy the old 60 Ft Dolls' song, *Love your hair* 'and everything below it'.

3/4 – Instant anxiety relief

One of the most helpful things I learned on my initial yoga therapy training is how brilliant moving our bodies is for anxiety relief. Movement honours the fight/flight impulse that it is usually inappropriate to act out in modern life. This stress response is triggered by all sorts of things. It lifts the sympathetic branch of the autonomic nervous system (ANS) **(22/10)** and starts a chain reaction throughout the body.

Our ancient ancestors mostly lived in parasympathetic mode **(9/1)**. The stress response was saved for genuine danger. Today, we're bombarded with 24/7 terrible 'breaking' news and are hyped up non-stop. Even an email or thought can trigger a cascade of stress hormones. Reading this sentence possibly isn't helping.

Fortunately, we can do things to minimise the negative impact. While not suggesting you run away from a stressful situation at work or punch the person who's irritating you, as soon as you can (maybe on your lunch break, maybe sooner), go for a brisk walk. Move. Burn off some of those stress hormones.

With 80 per cent of the signals going from body to brain **(29/2)** it makes sense to make the most of this. We can genuinely feel a sense of calm and peace instead of trying to force ourselves to 'calm down', which rarely works.

If you can't go for a walk, you might have space for a yoga mat so you can do some dynamic asanas like Sun Salutations. Even without a mat, Chair pose can be brilliant for using those larger muscles and getting us out of our ruminating minds and into our bodies. We don't have to do yoga. You might run or cycle or stamp your feet or do push ups. Whatever *you* want to do.

If you're unable to move physically, even *visualising* yourself being able to honour this natural impulse can bring some relief.

4/4 – Body scan with a twist

Body scans are brilliant for noticing how different parts of the body feel while not attempting to change anything; not torturing ourselves, but aiming to resist the urge to scratch or wriggle once we've begun as we can better cultivate the mind and actually change our experience.

Research, published in 2015 in the *Journal of Neuroscience* and *American Mindfulness Research Monthly*, showed how mindfulness meditations activate higher order brain regions. It doesn't just help us accept pain but actually reduces our experience of the pain.

As a twist to this body scan, pay close attention to each body part and to be curious about what each part may *need* from you. Instead of the usual attempts to override pain and other signals that are just pleas for self-care, really pay attention. How might you be extra kind to your ankles and so on?

For some parts, nothing beyond noticing physiological sensations may come up. For other more charged **(6/2)** parts, you may be surprised at what emerges.

5/4 – Brahmari

Also known as 'humming bee breath', Brahmari's mood boosting benefits may well be enhanced by the impossibility of taking ourselves seriously while practicing it.

Placing the thumbs gently in the ears, lick the lips. With them touching lightly, hum, maybe feeling the lips vibrate a little. Hum until the breath is completed then repeat, possibly higher or lower – traditionally, it's done at the same pitch but we can have fun, enhancing its playful benefits.

Research shows this increases theta brain wave activity (associated with meditation and relaxation). It also naturally elongates the exhalation **(9/1)**. As well as enlivening the system, research published in the *International Journal of Yoga* in 2014 found chanting Om **(22/1)** and Brahmari improves pulmonary function. It is also said to aid memory.

Yoga Journal published an article describing pain relief benefits when the sound and energy was sent to affected areas of the body numbed by pain. Brahmari can help with emotional pain, too, taking us out of our ruminating minds and into our bodies as we notice how each sound feels and where it vibrates.

Aim for 5-10 minutes but most of all, have fun with it.

6/4 – Ujjayi

This translates as 'victorious' and is brilliant for everyday use. As well as being able to use it for most yoga asana practice, we can go into it easily during stressful moments in our daily lives. As with all these practices, the more we do them when we're well, the more likely we'll be to remember them when we need them most.

With your mouth open and palm of hand in front so you can feel your breath, imagine yourself fogging up a mirror as you inhale and exhale, from the back of the throat. When you have a sense of this breath coming from the muscles we use to whisper, close the mouth and continue.

Ujjayi boosts parasympathetic activation **(9/1)** and helps us access higher states in meditation. It also activates the vagus **(29/2)** and helps control the mind. The sound as well as the feeling in the abdomen means there's more going on with Ujjayi - which some call Darth Vader breath and some Oceanic - so that helps us stay mindful.

Using Ujjayi breath makes entering the Relaxation Response **(1/1)** easier for most of us. It is believed to release GABA **(30/5)** calming the whole system.

7/4 – Alternative Nostril Breathing

A 1999 Czech Republic study using EEGs found that just five minutes of Alternative Nostril Breathing increased beta and alpha brain waves. Alpha waves are associated with being relaxed, creative and in touch with emotions. Beta waves are the kind we adults are usually in. It sounds paradoxical but shows the balancing nature of this breath.

Alternative Nostril Breathing can also help headaches and migraines, increase lung capacity and boost memory.

- ✓ Place the right thumb on the right nostril, inhale through the left before covering the left nostril with the right hand's fourth finger.

- ✓ Pause then release the thumb so you can exhale through the right nostril. You may want to place the index and middle fingers gently on the third eye.

It can sometimes ward off colds but if too blocked, simply visualising yourself doing this practice can help.

Repeat for 5-10 minutes (a shorter practice will still bring some benefits) aiming to keep a balanced breath (breathing in and out of each nostril the same length of time). If counting helps, do so (for example, in for four, out for four and so on – adapt the number to be comfortable for your breath rate).

When you finish, notice how you feel.

8/4 April – Dirga

This is brilliant for reminding ourselves that even when life feels overwhelming, we can create space with our breath.

Using your Ujjayi **(6/4)** if comfortable, or simply breathing from the lower lungs if not, breathe in three 'sips' of air and then exhale it all out. I initially felt stressed trying to make each sip equal but we don't have to worry about mathematical accuracy, just three sips in and one long exhalation **(9/1)**.

As with Ujjayi, Dirga gives us that extra focus, keeping the mind on our breath rather than our thoughts. It helps us create space in the lungs, fosters greater control of breath and improves lung capacity. Lynne Somerstein's research shows Dirga's benefits for anxiety. It is also used therapeutically for asthma and MS.

9/4 – Checking in with yourself

People often talk about the 'afternoon slump', recognising this widely known phenomenon yet still doing everything possible to power on through it. Sometimes, maybe on weekends, a nap might actually be possible. Other times, the idea may be laughable; our culture doesn't support siestas. Even so, honouring our bodies' natural cycles can help us not only feel more rested but be more efficient.

Some companies offer nap pods but it doesn't have to be an actual nap. It could be just taking any sort of downtime, maybe five minutes of your lunch or afternoon break to notice everything you can see, hear, smell and feel around you **(8/12)**. Maybe a Mindful Minute **(5/2)**.

Taking a little down time in the afternoon helps our systems come down naturally, it takes the edge of our stresses. We can then return to our work being more productive in the late afternoon as well as benefitting from a better night's sleep.

10/4 – Transference and countertransference

While these are therapeutic terms, transference and countertransference don't just happen in the consulting room. Have you ever taken an instant like or dislike to someone you just met? At an unconscious level, you may be transferring your feelings for someone else (an ex, old teacher, relative, whoever) onto this poor stranger and could be contaminating the relationship. Just by recognising, 'Oh! She/he reminds me of ___' makes it more conscious so we're less likely to act out.

Countertransference is also very powerful and mostly unconscious on both sides. We can get hooked into others' unconscious needs. For example, certain people may bring out our maternal or paternal sides. Or our Rescuer **(14/1)** (or Persecutor).

Again, realising that it may not be *our* feelings that we're feeling can help us notice rather than getting hooked in. Then we can make more conscious choices about how to be in each moment. Mindfulness and grounding **(13/3)** can help us notice when this happens.

11/4 – Cortisol releasing poses like lunge

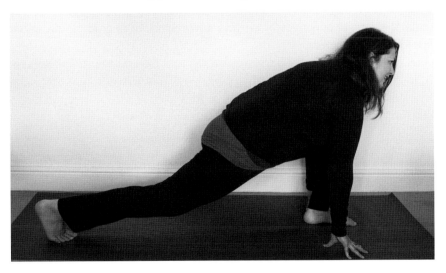

Sometimes, we wake up and have a good level of cortisol to help us get out of bed. Other times, we may have too much and feel anxious. On such mornings, we can release some of those excess stress hormones by doing some dynamic poses like Chair or a Lunge. Sun Salutations can be brilliant first thing in the morning but go with how you feel on any particular day. Warming up with gentler movement and poses helps us to avoid potential injuries.

12/4 – Willpower

Have you ever felt like you've simply run out of willpower? You're not imagining it. Studies show that the amount of choices we make before even leaving home in the morning can deplete our willpower stores for the day. We're using willpower to rise with our alarms rather than whenever we feel like getting up. Even choosing what to wear can drain this finite resource. Some people wear unofficial uniforms just to cut down on the time and energy consciously deciding what to wear takes.

Is there an area of your life in which you *know* what you need to be doing to progress towards your goals but are still not doing what needs to be done?

Whether it's to do with exercise, food, money or anything else, we can make it easier on ourselves by writing down what we're going to do, eat or spend the night before.

13/4 – Self-care audit

What's the first thing to go when life gets hectic? Sleep? Exercise? Meditation? Eating good food? Sex? Time with loved ones? Time alone? Time in nature? A clean (enough) home? Regular haircuts? Brushing your teeth? A massage?

We can do a quick self-care audit any time to help ourselves notice the signs earlier, staying as grounded and centred as possible. Even if that means saying 'No' to opportunities.

Think about a typical good (amp this up to wondrous if you like) day. List all the things you routinely do on such a day, from the moment you get up to bedtime.

You might want to print a copy out and stick it on the inside door of a cupboard you use daily. This can help you turn all these tiny, effortless actions when we're well and energised into everyday habits.

14/4 – The Ways

The Ways was one of my favourite modules during my psychosynthesis training.

In *Inevitable Grace: Breakthroughs in the lives of great men and women: guides to your self-realization*, psychosynthesis author (and co-founder of the organisation I trained at) Piero Ferrucci takes Assagioli's work on the Ways and runs with it.

Each Way is introduced from **15/4-21/4**. I recommend the book or working with a psychosynthesis therapist for more depth.

Some of our souls express themselves in this world through Beauty **(15/4)**, others through Action **(16/4)**, or Illumination (also known as Love) **(17/4)**, or Dance and Ritual **(18/4)**, or Science **(19/4)**, Devotion **(20/4)** or Will **(21/4)**.

Piero uses examples of genius in different areas (from Tolstoy to Isadora Duncan, Buddha and Patanjali, Mother Theresa to Mozart, Marie Curie to Galileo) to illustrate how we can better support our Selves **(21/8)** whichever Way (or Ways - sometimes, there's more than one we seek expression through) we most resonate with.

15/4 – The Way of Beauty

When we are awed by a beautiful sight in nature or piece of art, we're tuning in to this Way. For some, creating itself is an expression of this Way. Of course, we can be frustrated by the gaps between where we are and where we aspire to be. When I realised this was the Way for me, I stopped (mostly) giving myself a hard time for feeling so strongly about the desecration of nature, loud noises, litter and so on.

The soul's need for beauty, peace and harmony can be a brilliant creative driver. It can also lead us to potentially compromise ourselves for a more harmonious life. Creative types are often motivated by Beauty and Piero's examples include Anton Chekov, Van Gogh, Flaubert, Hector Berlioz, F Scott Fitzgerald, Simone de Beauvoir, Paul Gauguin, Petrarch, John Keats, William Wordsworth, Chang Tsao and Georgia O'Keefe.

How might you honour your soul's need for Beauty today?

16/4 – The Way of Action

Activists often come into this category, although there's overlap within categories and some identify with more than one. When we're on the Way of Action, we're concentrating on what needs to be done rather than thinking about the results. We're able to continue in spite of obstacles and hardships. We can also find freedom through practicing disciplines like yoga or a musical instrument.

It's about precision, respect, presence and service. Piero quotes from the *Baghavad Gita* where Krishna advises Arjuna to 'dedicate all actions to divinity'. Piero's famous examples include Albert Schweitzer, Florence Nightingale, Raoul Follerau, Mother Theresa, Mary Carpenter and Elizabeth Fry.

How might you honour your soul's need for Action today?

17/4 – The Way of Illumination (Love)

Also known as the Way of Love, people seeking self-actualisation on this path tend to be educators (liberating people's consciousness) and coaches, people who help us change our realities by changing our thoughts, seeing, 'love as a form of enlightenment'.

Concentration, reframing and introspection are elements of this way. Piero's 'geniuses in consciousness' include Buddha, Patanjali, Eckhart, Sankara, Hildegard of Bingen, St Teresa of Avila, Gopi Krishna, Sunryu Suzuki, Bertrand Russell and Tolstoy (here for his educational influence rather than literary legacy in Beauty).

How might you honour your soul's need for Illumination and Love today?

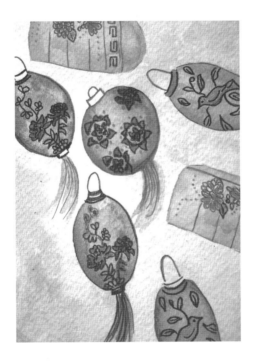

18/4 – The Way of Dance and Ritual

Apart from the overlap with sacred dance, this Way is about making the personal public through dance and rituals. It can include hatha yoga and Tai Chi as well as mime. Theatre comes under this Way. While we live in celebrity obsessed times now, Piero points out that throughout history, people have considered actors to be divine. They have access to different types of characters for different roles. No matter how familiar we become with our subpersonalities **(10/1)**, we don't inhabit them for months at a time on a film set or on stage.

Piero's examples include Al Huang Chiang, Isadora Duncan, Jean-Louis Barrault, Martha Graham and Black Elk.

How might you honour your soul's need for Dance and Ritual today?

19/4 – The Way of Science

This is all about 'the adventure of knowing', writes Piero. While each of the Ways requires resilience, perseverance and delayed gratification, the Way of Science takes this further. Honesty is a big part of this way. 'Maturity,' writes Piero, 'and perhaps enlightenment, consists in seeing reality as it is, even when it is at variance with our dearest hopes and most firmly held convictions.'

Piero's examples include Margaret Mead, Werner Heisenberg, Charles Sherrington, Einstein and Darwin.

How might you honour your soul's need to know something, for Science, today?

20/4 – The Way of Devotion

While many on this path devote themselves to whatever divinity they believe in, some devote themselves to other things like justice or money. When it's working well, people on this Way are filled with joy, love, passion and surrender. The flip side, of course, is fanaticism.

Piero's examples of geniuses of Devotion include Kabir, Rumi, Hafiz, St Teresa, St Catherine and St John of the Cross.

How might you honour your soul's need for Devotion today?

21/4 – The Way of the Will

This is the most dangerous and loneliest of Ways. Explorers and athletes push themselves beyond known boundaries, risk death and sometimes inspire us with their triumphs. A strong sense of Self can encourage us to keep going in spite of obstacles and discouragements.

As well as athletes and explorers, Piero counts Gandhi's risking his life to demonstrate non-violent direct action and people who ignored Nazi laws and rescued Jews and others from concentration camps. In spite of risks to themselves, people on this path follow their inner voice doing what needs to be done.

How might you honour your soul's need for this Way today?

22/4 – Showing appreciation to the earth

This Earth Appreciation Day, notice simple ways in which you can truly appreciate this wonderful organism that gives us all life. I'm drafting this in the garden with my bare feet enjoying the grass below - I just paused to lie down on my belly and surreptitiously hug the earth.

When we're on holiday, we tend to be in awe of our surroundings but the whole planet is pretty amazing. What do you appreciate most about your little corner of the world? How can you make it even more awesome **(5/12)**?

You might enjoy gardening or maybe picking up litter helps you; I have to be in the right mood so I'm picking it up with grace rather than secretly begrudging the people I consider to have no respect for the planet. Maybe a walk in nature **(31/7)**? Perhaps writing to your MP about an environmental issue that moves you to speak on behalf of the planet?

What might help you feel more appreciative of our planet today?

23/4 – Healthy blood pressure

This National Blood Pressure Day, you might want to take a moment to consider your own. Do you know if you're in the healthy range? Maybe you have high or low blood pressure? Get it tested - bearing in mind that many find it rises simply being tested.

What kind of action might you take? Finding a meditative practice you'll enjoy? Remember that yoga nidra **(9/3)** reduces blood pressure so can be great but it can bring on headaches with low blood pressure. Exercise that is fun? Eating healthier foods that don't feel like you're depriving yourself?

Maybe there is a person or situation in your life which, even without a blood pressure monitor, you can tell elevates your blood pressure. How might you tweak things so you're not so inflamed? It may mean reducing contact for a while until you find tools to manage your feelings around it.

24/4 – Resistance to guidance

It can be especially challenging to open up to guidance when we're feeling stressed and anxious and unable to take anything else on board. Opening up takes vulnerability. Most mornings, I use an open palmed mudra **(20/7)** to help me be especially open to guidance. Sometimes, the energy in my hands feels too intense and I'm unable to keep that open feeling.

Similarly, sometimes, in Tree pose **(16/11)**, I extend my branches - OK, arms. I know I'm not *really* a tree - and imagine myself opening up to the healing energy of the sun. Other times, it feels better to keep my hands in Prayer Position over my heart centre **(25/1)**.

Simply noticing how we feel when we ask for guidance can help us get into the flow of life more gently than forcing ourselves and possibly shutting down to good things in reaction.

If you feel open enough today, notice how it feels to visualise that shining light above you **(3/1)**, breathing in the sun's healing energies to awaken your potential.

25/4 – Happy DNA Day!

This DNA Day (there truly is a day for almost everything), we can notice our self-talk around DNA and what we know about the findings from the Genome Project.

How do we feel when we dismiss things as in our DNA? Does that inspire us to make healthy changes or does it leave us feeling defeated and hopeless? What about when we ponder the research around epigenetics? How our lifestyle changes can positively influence which genes literally turn on and off?

What would you do differently today if you believed you could positively influence your DNA?

If you're interested in having your DNA tested, visit <u>www.dnafit.com</u>

26/4 – More on mindfulness of the body

How have you noticed your thoughts about your body changing since you've become more mindful? Often, it can feel like it's making our self-loathing worse. This is rarely the case. We've just spent decades unconsciously telling ourselves these things. Mindful awareness makes it more conscious.

Noticing the thoughts we have about our bodies and other things is the first step towards changing them. Mindfulness is about acceptance. Simply accepting our feelings begins to shift them. It also helps us tune into our inherent resourcefulness **(15/10)**.

What changes feel good to make? What feels good to continue with? Which practices (so far) help you be more mindful of your body in a way that's good for your mind and heart, too?

27/4 – Moving and stretching

Waking up to see Rainbow MagnifiCat stretching and easing into her day helps me start the day well. Cats are brilliant at honouring what their bodies need and doing it. Being more mindful of our own bodies helps us notice that twinges, cramps, aches and pains are simply signals that we need to move or stretch differently to ease the pressure.

Pausing for a moment to scan your whole body, how would you most like to move and stretch right now? It may not be possible but there'll be *something* you can do in that direction to honour what your body needs.

28/4 – Inversions

Yoga poses that invert us include Headstand, Shoulder Stand **(2/5)**, Handstand, Down Dog **(30/4)** and Legs Up Wall **(29/4)**. Some fully invert us while with others, only part of us is upside down.

On earth, we spend most of our time upright. These upside down poses, in some ways, help us defy gravity (though not, like Elphaba in *Wicked*, in an able to fly sort of way). Just 3-5 minutes in an inversion helps fluid flow more effectively through veins, lymph channels, abdominal and pelvic organs. It makes it easier to absorb nutrients and flush toxins.

Anytime we're upside down, the circulatory system gets a bit of a break. The heart doesn't have to work so hard to pump blood back up from the feet. Inversions help us drain the fluids of the lower extremities as well as reducing congestion more effectively than sleep. It's important to ease into inversions: While many asanas are not our typical everyday human ways of sitting, standing or lying, inversions can put extra strain on the neck and spine if not done correctly.

Some women avoid inversions during menstruation but sometimes, it's fine. As with all yoga, we are all (men and women) best off paying attention to what feels friendliest for our own bodies on any given day.

29/4 – Legs Up Wall

This is the safest of all inversions. Awkward to get into but almost always worth the effort, this restorative pose helps pregnant women (or menstruating women who don't feel like inverting more strongly), people with high blood pressure, and those with injuries who can get several benefits from inversions without the potential risks.

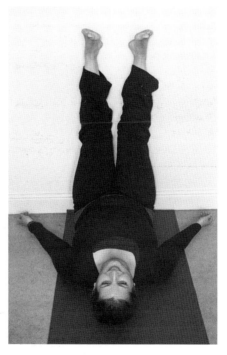

✓ Take the short end of your mat to a wall and bringing your buttocks as close to the wall as possible. Gently bring your legs around so you can straighten them up against the wall.

✓ Move the upper body so the head, neck and spine are comfortably aligned. Notice how it impacts your breath. How does it feel to have the support of the wall as well as the ground?

✓ If you want to, keeping the head and neck still, facing palms down alongside the body, bend the knees so the soles of the feet rest against the wall and give yourself a back massage. Inhale as you draw the body up off the mat and exhale as you gently bring it back down.

✓ Take as many complete breaths, inhaling up and exhaling down, as feels good then rest up against the wall again, noticing how you feel now.

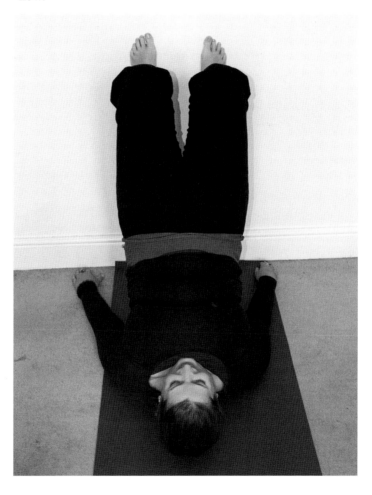

30/4 - Down Dog

- ✓ Downward Facing Dog or Down Dog is easy to come into from Table Top position (the neutral spine part of Cat/Cow **(16/8)**, with knees hip distance apart and hands either directly under or slightly in front of the shoulders). Aim to have the index fingers pointing forwards.

- ✓ Curl the toes under before lifting the knees and drawing your heels towards the mat.

- ✓ If there's a big gap, popping a folded blanket under the heels can offer more support. Looking back towards your knees, drop the shoulder blades so they (being upside down) go up.

- ✓ Aim for 3-5 full breaths here, noticing how easy or challenging it is to control the breath, maintaining your Ujjayi **(6/4)** or simple longer exhalation and full abdominal breath.

- ✓ To come out, either drop back to Cat/Cow or walk the feet towards the hands. Slowly fold up to standing.

Down Dog can help us tone the vagus nerve **(29/2)** and boost the ANS **(9/1)** as well as helping to stretch the sciatic nerve and supporting immune function.

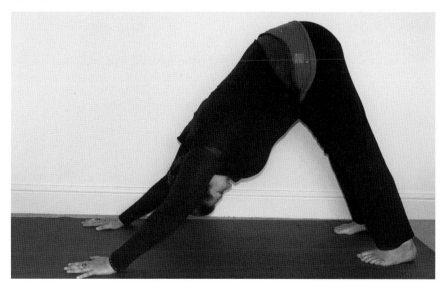

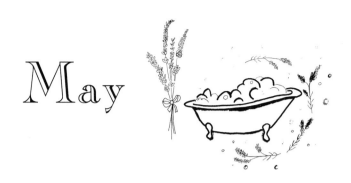

May

This month's tips include finding the learning in the setbacks, time travel, enhancing our lives and wellbeing with colour, mudras and how yoga naturally creates a hormone mimicked in drugs like Xanax.

1/5 – Beltane

This ancient festival of fertility, life and lust is a great time of year to contemplate what energises us and what we love. Also traditionally a day of promoting workers' rights, we can ask ourselves how we feel about the balance we have between what we feel we have to do and what we love to do.

As well as pondering our love lives and ways to bring more love into our lives overall, we can relax into the increasing warmth of the sun (in the UK) and notice the seeds we've planted so far and how they're growing.

2/5 – Shoulder Stand

- ✓ Shoulder Stand can be deceptively relaxing. If it feels good to ease into it today, start from Legs Up Against the Wall (**29/4**). After you've warmed up the spine with that gentle massage, as you inhale up again, draw the elbows toward the midline.

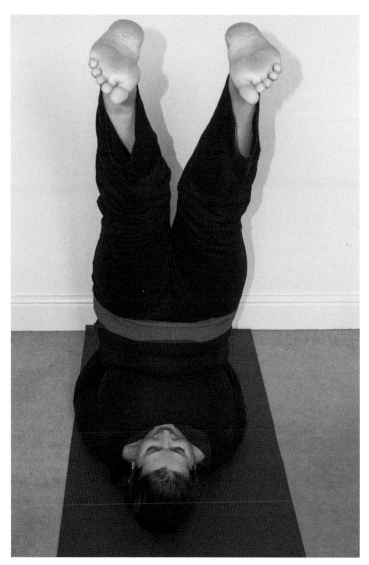

✓ Bring the hands to the lower back to support you as you aim the soles of the feet towards the ceiling.

✓ Notice the breath, aiming to continue with that longer exhalation **(9/1)** and full abdominal breath or your Ujjayi **(6/4)**. If it's comfortable to hold for five complete breaths, do so.

✓ Then come out either by taking Plough pose **(25/7)** or by bringing your legs back up against the wall.

3/5 – Mudras

Sometimes known as hand yoga, mudras are brilliant for directing energy (prana, charge, breath, life force and intention). When we're not in a place where it's appropriate to strike a yoga pose, we can support ourselves more subtly with one of these powerful gestures. Because they take so little energy and movement, we can do them when we're ill in bed. Or even surreptitiously at work or on the Tube - use your own judgment.

One of my favourite yoga teachers, Emma Turnbull (www.goddessyoga. co.uk) says she was taught them as 'psychic gestures. Yoga in your hands.'

The next few days (**4/5 to 7/5, 23/7 and 29/10**) introduce a few but there are many, many more.

Even on days we can't do a physical yoga practice, wellbeing can be literally at our fingertips.

4/5 – Chin mudra

Chin mudra involves touching the thumbs to the index fingers, with the rest of the hands open. Notice what naturally happens with your breath. Notice any other sensations.

We're all different but you may have noticed it helping to direct breath and energy into the abdomen and lower parts of the body. As well as supporting us in training this relaxing breath (**7/1**), Emma (**3/5**) points out that we can also consciously send prana, while using Chin mudra, to parts of the lower body that need some TLC: 'Anything from the naval down, including the abdomen, hips and legs.'

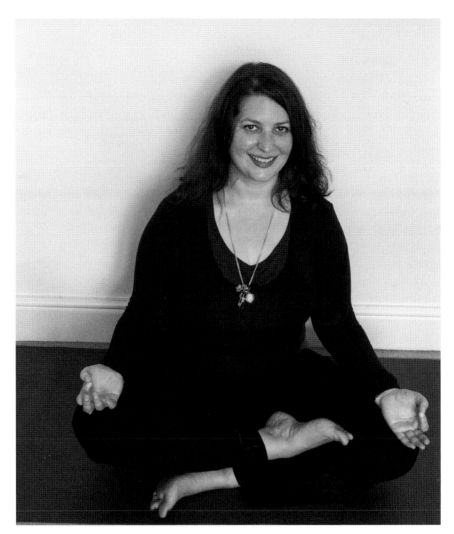

5/5 – Chinmaya mudra

Similar to Chin, here the last three fingers curl in and wrap up in the palm of the hand. 'It encourages thoracic breath **(3/3)** around the ribcage,' says Emma **(3/5)**. 'Chinmaya mudra can be used to send prana to the lungs, emotions, immune system, heart space and thymus.'

As with everything, notice how it feels for you.

6/5 – Adi mudra

This light fist is what newborn babies do: 'Open the palm of the hand,' says Emma, 'tucking the thumb into the palm and wrapping the other fingers around it. This encourages clavicle breath, a shallow breath under the collarbone. It brings energy up into the throat and head.'

Notice how you feel and, if you feel at all lightheaded or ungrounded, you can release this and go into your deeper, more grounding practices **(7/1)**.

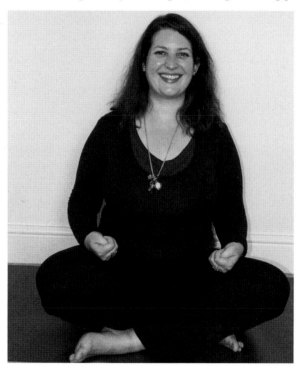

7/5 – Brahma mudra

Enclosing the thumbs as you make a first, turn the hands so they rest in your lap with the knuckles facing upwards.

'This is all about creation energy,' says Emma **(3/5)**. 'We can use it to send the energy around the whole body. It helps bring all three parts of the breath together for a complete yogic breath. It can bring a sense of deep peace and stillness.'

8/5 – NLP anchoring as mudras

I imagine that the originators of NLP were influenced by this ancient yogic practice when they encouraged people to use teeny tiny gestures (maybe touching an ear lobe) to anchor **(5/11)** specific states making it easier to access them when we need them most.

We can choose any small gesture that we wouldn't typically make as we relive the states we're anchoring. Maybe touching an earlobe or creating our own mudras with easy to replicate hand gestures. So, for example, if we're anchoring confidence, we can think of a time we've felt really at ease and confident in our own skin. As we make this memory vivid (using all our senses), use the tiny gesture.

Anytime we feel naturally confident, we can recreate the gesture to anchor the feeling more deeply. The more we practice, the stronger the new neural pathways will become. To strengthen it we can simply imagine ourselves feeling confident and do it. Waiting until we have the feeling can avoid anchoring *wanting* to be more confident.

Once it's properly anchored, simply recreating the gesture helps us access that actual sensation of feeling confident (or whatever you've chosen).

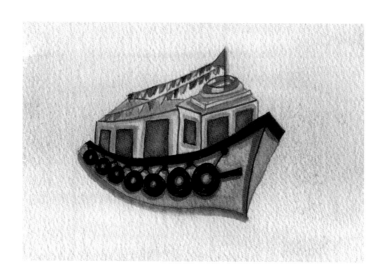

9/5 – Colour meditation

Wherever we look, we're surrounded by colour. Some landscapes are more soothing for our souls than others. We can't impact the weather but we can choose decorations, or at least accessories, for our surroundings. By being more conscious of the impact of colour on us, we can benefit in all sort of ways.

'We can use colour to nurture ourselves and improve all round wellbeing,' says Kath Roberts, a transformational coach (www.alchemy4 thesoul.com). Roberts uses colour a lot in her practice through Aura Color (similar to Aura Soma but with round bottles). She recommends playing with colour through what we wear, eat and drink, surrounding ourselves with colour and even visualising or meditating with colour.

'Visualise yourself breathing in a particular colour. For a fast and effective calming technique in a stressful situation, visualise the colour blue **(19/5)**. Visualise breathing in that blue calm, and breathing out red tension and relax.'

10/5 – Colourful clothing

Although I refused to wear anything but black as a teenager, my wardrobe is now filled with all the colours of the rainbow. It's been organised by chakra for more than fifteen years and I routinely choose what to wear not just for comfort and weather considerations but for how I want each item to help me feel.

Consider your clothing and accessories. What colours are you most drawn to?

When you consider your chakras **(16/7)**, maybe there are ways you can enhance (or balance) some by wearing more (or less) of a particular colour? We can also play with the KonMari approach **(19/3)** and hold each item, noticing which colours - and styles, of course - spark joy.

11/5 – Colours for decorating

Having lived in studio flats and other small spaces for much of my adult life, when I bought my first home, I painted it - according to chakras - the day I got the keys. Moroccan red and a beautiful burned orange for my bedroom, sunflower yellow for World HQ (my little home office), green for the kitchen and bathroom, royal blue for the living room and more green, this time darker, for the narrow hallway.

The following day, Feng Shui consultant Priya Sher (www.priyasher.com) visited and immediately told me most of it was wrong. Having looked forward to painting my own place for such a long time, I repainted within days. I followed her recommendations using white for the hallway, pale pink and pale yellow for the bedroom – like Battenberg and angel cake.

Years later, even though I'm still shocked at my now white bedroom, I sleep better than ever. While going white for the hallway, the bedroom was the biggest shock to *my* system (I'd always had colourful homes), you may find introducing splashes of colour as invigorating.

What colours would you like to experiment with? What feels like it might soothe your soul on a regular basis?

12/5 – Colour baths

More temporary than home décor or even clothing, adding colour to our bath water is a great way to check in with ourselves. How are we feeling? How would we *like* to feel? I started using food colouring in my bath water fifteen years ago. I initially just used a capful as I was worried about turning green - pre Elphaba. Over the decades, food colourings have become less strong so I use more. It's never stained the skin.

Because it's less public, we're less constrained by whether the colour will suit us or what others might think.

13/5 – Emotional duvets

Sometimes, we may know exactly what can help us feel better. Eating something nourishing rather than crisps for dinner? Going for a walk/run/some form of strong movement to use up those stress hormones and reduce that anxiety? And yet we resist.

On occasion, allowing ourselves to wallow can be healing. Joseph O'Connor's useful *NLP Workbook* (Thorsons, 2001) was, as NLP can be, very much about helping ourselves feel more dynamic, resourceful, excellent and so on. But my favourite page by far was where he acknowledged that sometimes, even though we *know* how to get ourselves into a more resourceful state **(15/10)**, we don't wanna. We want to wallow.

I have one bottle of black food colouring and rarely use it. But on such days, I consider running myself a black bath as part of the pity party I'm throwing myself. What helps you wrap yourself up in an emotional duvet? Not for every day but for those rare days when you just don't *want* to feel better?

14/5 – Red

Red is associated with the base (sometimes called root) chakra **(9/7)**. It can help us feel more safe, secure and grounded. Red is also said to promote courage, alertness, energy and present moment focus. It's a colour of empowerment and is also associated with love. Energising red can help us tap into our more resourceful selves **(15/10)** when life feels scary, especially concerning physical and financial safety.

Adding red to bathwater may sound like a bloodbath but I find it soothing and grounding. I often balance it with rose bubbles but sometimes add chilli chocolate bubbles depending on mood.

I remember an essay by Cynthia Heimel about wearing a 'symphony of reds'. While it was meant as a cautionary tale, I wear my own version of this whenever I need a boost. For other people, a red accent like a sock, tie, bag or lipstick may be more than enough.

15/5 – Orange

Associated with the sacral chakra **(10/7)**, orange can be a great reminder for us to slow down and enjoy all the good things life has to offer, from sex to a massage. From good, nourishing food to dance. Whatever feels good and life enhancing. Orange can help us tap into our personal power and self-worth. It's associated with movement, joy and dance. Some say it can help us digest life better and release self-pity. Also associated with creativity **(6/6)**, it can help us when we feel blocked. Orange can encourage us to go with the flow.

Orange baths can easily be created by mixing red and yellow. Ready mixed orange food colouring is often available now. I often complement this with Satsuma bubbles. Although I followed Sher's advice about wall colour **(11/5)**, I have plenty of red and orange accents.

16/5 – Yellow

This is associated with the Solar Plexus chakra **(11/7)** and can help us tap into our sense of personal power, even when that feels scary. Yellow has a cheerful, joyful energy, bringing warmth to our surroundings. Yellow is also associated with manifestation and money. Yellow can help us give and receive more. It's associated with successful new beginnings as well as the freedom to play. Some believe it strengthens the conscious mind so can aid focus.

A yellow bath may sound a bit grim but with lemon bubbles, this is one of my favourites.

Again, play with the shades you like the most.

17/5 – Green

One of my favourite colours, green is associated with the heart chakra **(25/1 and 12/7)** compassion, love, healing, regeneration, energy, growth, harmony, peace and even money. Because the heart chakra is where the lower and upper chakras come together, green is associated with balance and integration. It can also help us accept ourselves as we are rather than how we wish we were.

As well as adding green to our bathwater, painting certain walls, adding accents and wearing green can be great reminders to open our hearts and take better care of ourselves.

As with everything, you know yourself best. How do you feel about green? What are your favourite and least favourite shades? Does learning more about the heart chakra make you want to include more (or less)?

18/5 – Pink

Also associated with the heart chakra **(25/1** and **12/7)**, we can use pink when we need a reminder to be gentle with ourselves. Hot pinks can encourage us to be a bit bolder. Pink is also associated with releasing worries, pure spiritual energy, happiness, joy, laughter and peace. It's said to help increase self-compassion, helping us accept and release our faults so we can get on with life.

I use a little red when I want a pink bath and often mix it with rose bubbles.

If it weren't for the past several years' didactic 'pink for girls and blue for boys' marketing, I'd probably like pink much more.

19/5 – Blue

Associated with the Throat chakra **(13/7)**, some people report that even wearing a blue scarf aids their communication skills. Especially when they need to speak up for themselves or give a presentation. Pale blue or turquoise are especially good but, again, go with your favourite shades. This is for *you*. Blue is also associated with peace, relaxation, wisdom, truth, integrity and openness. It is believed by some to stop nightmares.

Every shade is calming, soothing and restful. Blue can help us express ourselves better and do so in a gentle but still powerful way.

I often add lavender bubbles to my blue baths and typically have them later in the day as they're more calming.

20/5 – Purple

Purple is associated with the Third Eye chakra **(14/7)** and we can use it in our décor, clothing and for baths (mix red and blue) when we want to honour and encourage our intuition and inner wisdom, dreams, intellect and understanding. It has regal associations, too, so can feel empowering in an Activating Inner Queen or King **(17/1)** way.

Purple is also associated with the intangible and mysterious. It is considered to be useful for meditative, psychic and healing work. Purple is said to help with headaches and hair issues as well as being a colour of transformation.

Great before bed, again, play with the shades you love the most (from rich regal purple to lilac).

21/5 – Other colours

White and gold are often associated with the Crown chakra **(15/7)**. They can help us tune into our connection with the Divine in whatever form we understand that to be.

Then of course there's trusty black. Great for more than looking svelter, black is traditionally associated with helping to keep negativity at bay.

Metallic colours like rose gold, silver and bronze can help us feel a little more sparkly.

Sequins, sparkles, tweeds and other fabrics of course change the associations of items. As do patterns. Do you like bold geometrics? Florals?

As with everything, notice your own associations and feelings with each colour and build up your own resources **(15/10)** around your favourites.

22/5 – Time travel to help Younger You(s)

When we think back over our lives so far, we can often be harsh, blaming our inner child or younger selves for not x, y or z-ing. But we were doing the best we could at the time.

When one of my psychosynthesis trainers talked about a younger part of himself who hadn't made great decisions, he smiled, explaining it was part of his journey. I remember hoping that I might come to view my own Drunken Mess (as I called one of my own younger selves at the time) with even a fraction of that compassion instead of the self-loathing I felt at not having taken better care of myself for so many years.

Fortunately, we can all go back in time (in our imaginations, at least) and send a little love and compassion to ourselves at any age we have issues around. Digging out old pictures can help* us hone in on certain times of our lives. By giving our younger selves the care they needed back then, we help heal our whole selves.

---

* with trauma, this can be a painful process. Wait until you're ready or work with a good therapist.

23/5 – Smaller increments of time travel

While we can view key events in our lives (so far) overall **(22/5)**, we can also take smaller steps and think back over the last few hours. It's easy to think of all the things we wish said in certain situations. I've often wished I had Aaron Sorkin (*The West Wing, Studio 60 on the Sunset Strip* and *The Newsroom*) or Shonda Rhimes **(14/2)** scripting my dialogue in real life.

Instead of letting these thoughts whir, beating ourselves up for not being amazingly articulate when we were stressed about a particular meeting, conversation or other situation we 'should' have handled better, we can send these slightly younger selves a little hug instead.

Immediately, that amygdala alarm bell part of the brain is soothed by the more sophisticated prefrontal cortex. It reassures us that even though we weren't perfection personified – after all, we're human - it's all good.

24/5 – More hugs for younger you(s)

In a similar vein, you may want to send some healing hugs towards younger yous which don't necessarily stand out as particularly messed up (pre compassionate, 'Part of the journey'). We can flip through old photo albums, love letters, diaries and other mementos, sending mental hugs to ourselves at all the ages that crop up.

How does it feel to hug your younger selves at 39, 16, 6 or even as a newborn?

Can you feel the shift in energy in yourself today? The more we can accept ourselves as much as possible, the better able we are to take good care of ourselves now and in the future.

25/5 – Happy International Day of Happiness!

When you hear that today's an International Day of Happiness, does it make you smile?

What are your associations with happiness?

For many, happiness is too big an energy. It can feel like pressure. All emotions are fleeting. We can create as much stress in trying to attain and maintain happiness as we might by trying to suppress perfectly normal 'negative' emotions like anger and sadness.

Today, why not let ourselves of the hook and just allow ourselves to feel however we actually feel? No expectations. No pressure. As little judgment as our judgypants human minds allow.

Instead, we can notice the times we naturally smile or laugh or feel happiness in all its guises. Let it creep up on us instead of trying to hunt it down.

26/5 – The learning is *in* the setbacks

I've heard various forms of it all being 'Grist to the mill', 'It's all data' and the NLP presupposition of 'No such thing as failure, only feedback'. Nora Ephron was famously raised by her writer parents to know 'Everything's copy'. She later turned her divorce and other heartaches into blockbuster films as well as personal essays.

My BACP Coaching colleague and friend, Gill Fennings-Monkman MBE (www.counsellingforachange.com) takes it even further saying 'The learning is *in* the setbacks'. She talks about greeting dismayed tales of falling off various wagons by her clients with an enthusiastic and curious, 'Great! Let's look at what happened. Let's get curious about your experience with kindness.'

When we're able to explore setbacks with compassion and curiosity **(7/6)** instead of beating ourselves up about them, we can learn from them.

Soothing ourselves instead of adding more stress to the situation can help us potentially use the data – however upsetting it may feel in the moment - to spark a growth spurt in whichever area(s) we're struggling with.

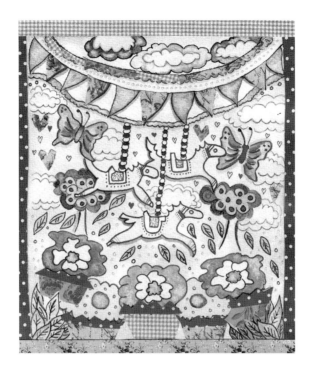

27/5 – 'And what would happen if you *did* disturb your cat?'

Another BACP Coaching colleague and friend, Michèle Down (<u>www.micheledowndynamics.co.uk</u>), made me cry with laughter with this compassionate but bemused response. I'd been explaining how I would regularly contort myself around my sleeping Rainbow MagnifiCat to avoid disturbing her. I put my cat's sleep ahead of my own.

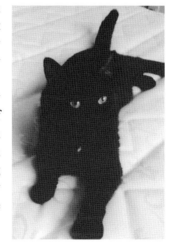

All that *would* happen is that Rainbow would sigh (in my imagination) and jump off the bed (in reality). I still sometimes stay in uncomfortable positions to avoid that but laugh (quietly, so as not to disturb her) remembering Michèle's words and expression. It's my choice. Awareness almost always brings more choice.

Can you think of an area in your life where you believe something which isn't necessarily true? Checking in with ourselves and following through on what we think might happen if we do (or don't do) something can help us regain perspective.

Of course, we might *still* choose to carry on putting our cats' comfort ahead of our own (or your equivalent situation), on occasion.

28/5 – Amnesty International Day

While Amnesty International (www.amnesty.org) works tirelessly on behalf of people around the world who need an amplified voice, we can all take today to heart. As well as checking out their work and getting involved if so moved, it's a great day to let ourselves out of the prisons in our mind. What might we declare an amnesty around in our own lives? How can we let ourselves off the hook for not handling something perfectly or even differently?

How can we move forward, having learned from the experience but no longer torturing ourselves about it?

The more compassion we can learn to show ourselves, the more compassionate we can be with others.

29/5 – Yin breath practice

I learned this Daoist breath practice from transformational relationship coach, Elena Angel (www.elenaangel.com):

✓ Breathing in and out through the nose, when you have exhaled completely, sigh, making a sound 'haaaaa' with open mouth.

- ✓ As you make this sighing sound, you may notice that the navel is pushed back towards the spine. Allow it to pop out again when you inhale, keeping the belly soft. Notice how much more space there is for air to stream into your body through your nose.

- ✓ With each exhalation notice where the sound is vibrating in your body. Each breath is an invitation for the sound to reach deeper, all the way down to the sex. Remain mindful of sensations, emotions and thoughts as they arise. Stay with the breath and the vibration of the sound.

- ✓ As the vibration moves further down in your body, you might hold more specific intentions, focusing your attention and feeling into that loving intention towards yourself and your body. Coming to the heart, experience feelings of tenderness, joy, compassion and your most heartfelt desires. Reaching deeper into the belly, feel your emotional depth, your powerful core, a feeling of safety, presence, nourishment, wholesomeness, stability, connection with the Earth, your natural wisdom and anything else that may be there. Breathing down to the sex, feel your aliveness, creativity, playfulness, sexiness, sensuous pleasure and anything else that may be there. Smile inside.

- ✓ Practise this style of breathing at any time, for as long as feels comfortable. It is often useful to loosen the joints, shake and stretch any parts of the body that feel like they're holding tension. If emotions arise, breathe through them. Notice particular sensations when you have reached the genitals/perineum. Continue to breathe through feelings for as long as you like. Maintain a loving intention and attitude of acceptance.

- ✓ Keep a sense of downward flow: energy/breath flowing in and down and through, like water cascading down.

30/5 – GABA

Boston University Medical School researcher Dr Chris Streeter, (working with McLean Hospital's Dr Eric Jensen, among others) discovered that just one hour's yoga practice increases GABA levels. GABA (gamma-amino butyric acid) is the brain's primary inhibitory neurotransmitter. Drugs like Prozac mimic its relaxing effects. As well as lowering stress and anxiety and improving mood, by boosting GABA levels through yoga, the only side effects we risk are added flexibility, strength, stamina and wellbeing.

While she's not recommending yoga *instead* of medication, the research shows how effective a complementary therapy it can be for stress and anxiety issues.

You can watch an interview with Dr Streeter here https://www.youtube. com/watch?v=asRPQ6mWZUg

31/5 – Universal strengths

Assagioli created psychosynthesis over a hundred years ago. While he was as interested in people's potential as their wounding, it's really only in the last few decades that 'positive psychology' has taken off. Martin Seligman and his colleagues have been studying what makes people happy and fulfilled so we can all learn from these effective strategies for living well.

I learned about Universal Strengths (characteristics that are viewed positively throughout the world) from Bridget Glenville-Cleave. The author of *Positive Psychology: A Practical Guide* talked about qualities such as Awe, Authenticity, Bravery, Citizenship, Creativity, Curiosity, Fairness, Forgiveness, Gratitude, Hope, Humility, Humour and playfulness, Integrity, Kindness, Leadership, Love, Open-mindedness, Persistence, Prudence, Self-control, Social intelligence, Spirituality, Vitality and Wisdom.

Over the next few days **(2/6-12/6)** and through the rest of the year **(14/6, 18/6-20/6, 22/6-24/6, 11/9, 27/10, 14/11, 3/12, 5/12** and **7/12)** we'll take a closer look at each. We'll explore how they benefit us when in balance as well as how each can be overplayed or underplayed.

June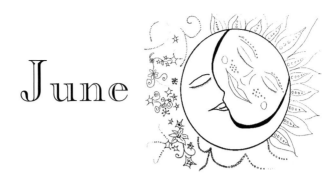

This month's tips include shame and vulnerability, ways to boost our will, some of the universal strengths identified in positive psychology and turning pain into life-saving movements.

1/6 – International Children's Day

In an ideal world, every child on the planet would know they mattered. All would be safe, sheltered, educated and fed and watered (I love that the Welsh word for child is plant). It's easy to feel helpless when we hear about child refugees not only having endured horrors but being denied care having survived. Similarly, there may be children in our own families and neighbourhoods we feel need more care and security.

To honour International Children's Day, we can notice what, in our world, we can do to make things better for a child or some children. It may be taking some kind of environmental action to safeguard the planet's future for them. Or it may be babysitting for a loved one's little ones, doing something extra special for your own, volunteering, fundraising or donating money to a children's charity close to your heart like www.unicef.org.

Maybe it's simply doing something to honour your own inner child **(22/5)** or taking Child pose **(28/10)**. What feels good for you today?

2/6 – Playfulness

I met a friend in the pool after my swim yesterday. Having done my usual 'proper' swim, I had five minutes before she was due so instead of my usual (space permitting) quick handstand and floating before cursory spa and steam, I lost count of the number of underwater handstands I did. As I floated, an older man laughed at me saying, 'Don't work too hard!' and I told the stranger I'd already swum for an hour. On reflection, I was prouder of myself for the playful handstands and floating than the routine swims I adore but which don't fall under 'play'.

When the universal strength **(31/5)** of playfulness is in balance, we can access our flow and creativity **(6/6)** more easily. It's energising and invigorating. Fun!

If we overplay it, we may lack purpose **(7/12)** and fulfilment. We might annoy those who feel resentful that they work while we play.

When we underplay playfulness, life can become very dull. We can become prone to burnout.

By noticing the kinds of things that help us tune into this quality (like Improv **(26/6)**), we can (I know, it's like scheduling spontaneity) be more playful on purpose.

How might you be more playful today?

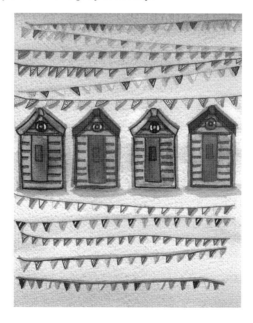

3/6 – Authenticity

Authenticity is one of those words that often elicits groans. Really, it's just about letting our true colours show. Being ourselves. When it's in balance, we're able to become (to quote Oprah) our 'best selves'. But it's not just about being our best. When we're truly authentic, we're able to express and allow ourselves to feel *whatever* we're feeling.

We're naturally inspired by the people we see being *their* whole selves, out of whichever closets life may have tried to keep them in. Similarly, us being *our*selves can inspire others to be more themselves. People like David Bowie, Lady Gaga and Grace Jones turn it into an art form.

When overplayed, we might forget that others' feelings matter as much as our freedom of expression. When underplayed, we might fail to speak up for ourselves, dressing, saying and doing what we think others will approve of. Slowly dying on the inside.

How might you be more authentic today?

4/6 – Bravery

We can easily see how bravery is considered a universal strength **(31/5)**. When it's in balance, we can change the world by being brave enough to stand up for ourselves and others.

When we overplay it, we might become too fond of throwing caution to the wind and risk our (and even others') safety for nothing.

Underplayed, we might forget our resourcefulness and cower in the face of challenges instead of stepping up.

Poses like Warrior II **(20/2)** can help us with this balance.

How might you be braver today?

5/6 – Citizenship

When we're conscious of our connection to others in our neighbourhoods, countries and the world at large, we make decisions that benefit beyond just our own lives. The Native American tradition of the Children's Fire, where Elders considered the impact of their decisions on the lives of future generations is a great example of this.

When in balance, citizenship helps us remember our social responsibility, we're loyal. We can be team players.

Overplayed, we might forget our own needs for the sake of the group. We might also feel the weight of the world on our shoulders without making any difference in terms of social responsibility. We might be loyal to a fault. Excessive patriotism and fundamentalism can be examples of citizenship being overplayed.

Underplaying it can lead to feelings of disconnection, that nothing we do matters. Having little or no regard for the consequences of our behaviours on others.

How might you be a good world citizen today?

6/6 – Creativity

When our creativity is in balance, it energises us. It can help us find solutions to impossible seeming situations. It can help us create art, music, business ideas and even babies.

Overplayed, we might blur the lines and lie to ourselves and others. We might also overdo it, forgetting to 'refill the well' as Julia Cameron, bestselling author of the *Artist's Way* advises. We might burn out.

Underplayed, we may feel that life's a bit grey and lack the inspiration to make the tweaks and changes that can transform our experiences.

How might you be honour your creativity today?

7/6 – Curiosity

Recognising this as my #1 strength during Glenville-Cleave's **(31/5)** workshop was transformative. I could see how, in balance, my curiosity is brilliant for my work (both at Feel Better Every Day and with my writing). When I overplay it, I say 'Yes' to too much. I spread myself too thin.

When our curiosity is in balance, we're engaged with life and learning. It can help us connect not just with ourselves and loved ones but people from all over the world. A curious and compassionate approach to our own foibles is incredibly healing.

Overplayed, we might veer towards nosiness or even danger - they say it killed the poor cat. Underplayed, we can become myopic and insular.

How might you be more curious today?

8/6 – Fairness

Fairness helps us live harmoniously, contributing and taking in appropriate measure. From early childhood, we *know* when something's not fair. Injustice, people getting away with bad behaviour, others being exploited, being punished just for being themselves … even typing this, I can feel my blood pressure rise. (Time for a Mindful Minute **(5/2)**.)

Overplayed, we can live our lives as irritating class prefects, constantly policing the world around us.

Underplayed, we might forget that we're all connected and take shortcuts which help us but potentially (or even obviously) harm others.

How might you be more fair today?

9/6 – Forgiveness

Forgiveness is a wonderful thing. I often think that if we could take all the troubled spots of the world and, instead of calling them the names they go by and getting hooked into traumatic histories on all sides, if we could just say A and B and start fresh, people on all sides could heal and, in time, forgive.

When forgiveness is in balance, we're able to rise above things.

Overplayed, we might work so hard at forgiving others for what we're not yet ready to forgive, it could be harmful to ourselves. A betrayal. When this feels like the case, we can practice forgiving ourselves for not being saintly enough to genuinely feel that complete forgiveness. We can also forgive ourselves for our part in whatever the situation.

Underplayed, we can hold grudges for decades. Apart from the health risks, this kind of attitude depletes joy and feeds bitterness.

How might you be more forgiving today?

10/6 – Gratitude

Study after study (including Wong, YJ et al.'s 2016 research around gratitude writing alongside psychotherapy, published in *Psychotherapy Research*) shows the benefits of gratitude on our wellbeing.

When in balance, we naturally pause to notice the beautiful smell of the roses or whatever delights the days offer.

Overplayed, we might feel indebted to others, undeserving.

Underplayed, we stop noticing all the blessings in our lives. Our focus on lack can make us feel disheartened.

No matter what's going on, we can pause and mentally list five things, right now, we're grateful for. This helps us access more of our resources enabling us to deal with the things we were stressing about as well as bringing a sense of graciousness to our lives. Some people take it further with gratitude journals (Sarah Ban Breathnach's *Simple Abundance* helped

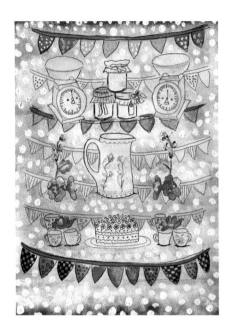

popularise this practice in the 1990s) but even just a moment, pausing in appreciation can shift our perspective.

How might you be more appreciative today?

11/6 – Hope

Hope is one of the positive emotions that can help us increase dehydroepiandrosterone (DHEA) levels **(2/12)**. When we have hope, we can endure more. We can draw on our resources. We can feel the pleasure of anticipating even more goodness in our future.

When we overplay hope, we may leave too much to chance. Hoping for the best isn't a great strategy without practical steps.

Underplayed, we can find ourselves in the depths of despair, as Anne of Green Gables might have said. Without hope, everything can feel futile. Hopeless.

How might you honour hope in your life today?

12/6 – Humility

When humility is in balance, we're able to acknowledge our achievements in a matter of fact but understated manner. We're not seeking approval and we're not diminishing our efforts.

Overplayed, humility may mean missing out. We don't have to blow our own trumpets to deafening and irritating degrees. But we *can* learn to speak up for ourselves and step into our power more.

Underplayed, of course, we can be pretty unpleasant to be around. Boasting, showing off and being arrogant.

How might you honour your humility today?

13/6 – Burmese meditation technique for mindfulness of thoughts

I learned this during my initial yoga therapy training. It's a great way to get beyond the content of our thoughts to truly notice what's going on for us. Spending even a few minutes categorising our thoughts can help us cultivate the mind:

Analysing helps us make sense of things. Sometimes, we overanalyse and get stuck.

Imagining is essential not just for creative endeavours but for transforming our lives by imagining better. We might misuse our imaginations by catastrophising.

Judging is great for making decisions and filtering information. Often, we can judge ourselves and others too harshly.

Worrying is another misuse of imagination. Even though we're wired to see danger, by simply noticing when we're worrying, we can step back.

Planning is essential for getting things done but sometimes, we can get so future focused, we forget to be present.

Doubting is helpful when it comes to not being gullible. Too much doubt makes us cynical.

Remembering can help us draw strength and joy from the past. Too much nostalgia can make us feel like foreigners in the present.

Simply noticing the kind of thought rather than getting sucked into the thought itself can be both challenging and restful for the mind.

Which kind of thought do you notice yourself having most frequently right now?

14/6 – Humour

Often paired with playfulness **(2/6)**, when humour is in balance, we're able to enjoy life's absurdities. Laughing helps us get through tough situations. We can even defuse explosive situations. People like nurses and firefighters are known for their gallows humour as they're dealing with the unthinkable and need some lightness.

Overplayed, we might depend on it too much **(15/1)** or put our need for a laugh ahead of someone else's need for dignity. Often powerful groups use 'Where's your sense of humour?' or 'It's just banter' to keep minorities down.

Underplayed, we may act as if we've had a sense of humour bypass. We start taking ourselves and things too seriously.

How might you honour your sense of humour more today?

15/6 – The Will

Although psychosynthesis is a transpersonal psychology, its creator, Roberto Assagioli, was very clear on the essential need for the will. The will helps us get things done. Strong Will helps us power through. Skilful Will helps us discern the best approach to take. Good Will helps us consider others. And Transpersonal Will helps us 'Let go and let God' (Goddess, the Universe or whatever you believe in).

Assagioli's will helped him endure imprisonment during World War II. How might you hone your different types of will today?

16/6 – Will boosting exercise

In Assagioli's treatise on the will, *The Act of Will,* one of the will boosting exercises he recommends is standing one legged on a chair each day. His idea is that we commit to *something* and do it no matter what. Personally, I didn't try this but have, in recent years, made my daily meditation and yoga* non-negotiable. Not in a punitive way but I know how much better off I am since using my will to make them habitual.

We can all choose something we're going to do no matter what. Maybe it's flossing our teeth or taking a multivitamin. Choose something small and build up. Notice how it feels to develop more will in this area and how it impacts other areas of your life.

17/6 – Evocative words

Assagioli recommended writing down the qualities we want to develop so we'd see them regularly and be more motivated to use our will. I visited Assagioli's house in Florence for a few years ago. It was humbling to see his own evocative words on display, 'Pazienza' (patience) and 'Serenita'

---

* Some days it's a 'proper' practice. Other mornings, maybe just one or two asanas. Maybe even 'just' Child pose **(28/10)**. The act of will is getting onto the mat and noticing what feels best for my body each morning

(serenity) having encouraged him. Both are qualities I struggle with but had assumed he had in spades.

We can use any kind of paper. We can type, use calligraphy or simply scrawl our evocative words. I like bathroom crayons, writing them on bathroom tiles so I'm reminded of the qualities I want to enhance several times a day.

18/6 – Integrity

When our integrity is in balance, we keep our word to ourselves and to others. We can be counted on. We do the 'right thing' whether or not anyone else is watching.

Overplayed, our inner Judgypants **(10/1)** can come out. We become incredibly hard work and others probably feel less inclined to do (our perception of) the 'right thing'.

Underplayed, we're acting dishonestly. We might feel like we're getting away with it at some level but lying (especially to ourselves) rarely feels good.

How might you honour your inherent integrity more today?

19/6 – Self-control

When our self-control is in balance, we're literally more in balance. We're able to put immediate pleasures aside in order to reap the benefits of waiting. We're better able to think of the common good rather than thinking only of ourselves.

Over-played, self-control can make us beyond boring. *We* might be fascinated by how little we're eating/ drinking/smoking or how much we're exercising and so on. But it's rarely entertaining for others to hear about. They're also likely to hear our self-control as judging their lack.

Underplayed, self-control can make us feel like our whole lives are spinning out of control. Whether it's spending, eating, drinking, drugging, lying or whatever else in excess, we can easily spiral into shame **(27/6)** rather than gently bringing ourselves back on track.

How might you hone your self-control today?

20/6 – Leadership

When leadership is in balance, be it in our homes, workplaces, communities or organisations, we inspire others to step up. We empower others. Leadership is also important if the only person we're leading is ourself. Are we being a good leader? Have we perhaps ceded control to a less helpful subpersonality **(10/1)**?

Overplayed it, we might become bossy, attempting to bully others into our way of doing things.

Underplayed, we might feel helpless. As Alice Walker so beautifully put it, 'The most common way people give away their power is by thinking they don't have any.'

How might you honour your inner leader more today?

21/6 – Summer Solstice

This longest day of the year (in this part of the hemisphere) is also known as Litha. It's a great time of year to celebrate and thank Mother Earth. We can lie on the ground and breathe in its healing energy. It's also about giving thanks and counting our blessings.

Litha is a useful time to consider our contribution to the world, contemplating our 'public self'. Getting really grounded, knowing we have that nourishing, nurturing support below us, guiding our every step, we can let ourselves dream big.

How would you most like to contribute your skills, talents and gifts to make the world a better place?

22/6 – Social intelligence

Social intelligence helps us read a room and adapt. We balance who we are with where we are, what we're doing and who we're with.

Overplayed, we might forget ourselves and focus too much on others' reactions. We might become manipulative.

Underplayed, we may forget ourselves, being inappropriate for the place and people around us.

Having said that, Amy Cuddy **(26/11)** found that some less socially intelligent people did *better* in presentations. They weren't put off their work by body language and other cues from listeners.

How might you enhance your social intelligence today?

23/6 – Open-mindedness

When in balance, open-mindedness helps us hear others' viewpoints and make an informed decision. We can, as the pre-Presidential Barack Obama told Oprah Winfrey, 'disagree without being disagreeable.' An open mind can help appreciate new ideas.

Overplayed, while our brains are unlikely to actually fall out, we can perhaps forget common sense in favour of listening too intently to obvious nonsense. It might also make us very indecisive as we're so able to see the benefits of different approaches we fail to make a decision.

Underplayed, we risk fundamentalism and didactic approaches which rarely end well for anyone concerned.

How might you be more open-minded today?

24/6 – Persistence

Another Universal Strength **(31/5)**, persistence is essential in many areas. Without persistence, almost nothing worthwhile would have been accomplished. Even when people seem to have conjured up magic, effortlessly writing a sublime book or spectacular song, painting a masterpiece or stumbling across a breakthrough scientific discovery, their previous efforts have created the conditions for this burst of divine inspiration. Inherently, we all want to grow and develop. Toddlers don't give up when their first steps land them back on the floor. But as we get older, we often beat ourselves up more for not reaching perfection with our initial efforts.

Overplayed, we might refuse to take no for an answer and make unwanted advances or worse. We might also continue down a path without adapting our approach and learning from our 'failures'.

Underplayed, we just give up. Depriving ourselves and, potentially, the world, of all we have to offer.

How might you balance persistence today?

25/6 – Ovulation

This summery, full lunaresque energy brings a sense of 'I can do anything,' says Lisa Lister, author of *Code Red* **(28/2)**. Oestrogen and testosterone peak leaving us feeling more confident, active, powerful and extraverted. While ovulation is typically associated with fertility and pregnancy, it's a time for all of us to tap into our creativity **(6/6)**. No babies required. We can use this energy to be productive, making time for projects that are meaningful for us and generally enjoying a sense of ease as we flow through life.

It's a great time for manifesting so we can get clearer on our intentions. We can charge them with the energy we have for practical action too. By dusting off our vision boards **(24/12)** and sankalpas **(9/3)**, we can ensure they represent what we want for ourselves now.

26/6 – 'Yes, and …' improvising at life

At school, a drama teacher encouraged me to do more Improv but I was far too self-conscious and disembodied to go for it. I preferred scripts. Certainty. While I read of shy souls turned megastars finding themselves in their roles, I was never able to forget my self-consciousness enough to overcome routine stage fright. Looking back, I was having panic attacks aged 13 but I didn't know what they were. Just thought they would kill me. So dramatic.

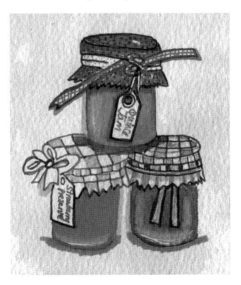

Years later, reading memoirs by the likes of Tina Fey and Amy Poehler and seeing them and others on James Lipton's *Inside the Actors Studio*, I so loved what they all said about Improv creating a 'Yes, and …' approach to life as well as the scenes, I decided to try it.

Essentially, it's about agreeing with what is and building on it; acceptance and creativity **(6/6)**. While the classes I attended, with Steve Roe of Hoopla fame (www.hooplaimpro.com) were terrifying initially, they helped me truly understand the concept of mindfulness and being in the moment. They also remain amongst the most valuable trainings I've done in terms of helping me approach life and work more playfully **(2/6)**.

Steve and his colleagues teach Improv skills to business people as well as standup comedians and others. '"Yes, and …" is especially helpful in creative meetings,' says Steve. 'The next time someone suggests an idea, try saying "Yes, and…" then building on their idea rather than saying "No" or "But" and rejecting it. "Yes, and …" enables us to play and build upon ideas while delaying judgement, so the group can collaborate together and discover new ideas together.'

27/6 – Brené Brown on shame and vulnerability

If you haven't already seen Dr Brené Brown's groundbreaking talks on shame and vulnerability (and how essential they are if we want to live full, wholehearted lives), you can view them below.
https://www.ted.com/talks/brene_brown_on_vulnerability?language=en
https://www.youtube.com/watch?v=psN1DORYYV0

Simply noticing, 'Ahh, Shame Spiral!' is brilliant in terms of avoiding being sucked in fully. Once we're conscious of what's going on, we can reach out for support. This needs to be appropriate as we don't want to compound our shame by opening up to someone who can't handle it.

The bestselling author's books include *Rising Strong, Daring Greatly, The Gifts of Imperfection, Power & Vulnerability* and *I Thought it was Just Me (But it Isn't)*.

28/6 – Eve Ensler and shame

Long before I came across Brené Brown, Eve Ensler's *The Vagina Monologues* was life changing for me. Especially V-Day (www.vday.org), the movement it inspired in an effort to fund grassroots organisations working to end violence against women and girls. When I met Ensler and Gloria Steinem at a V-Day conference in New York in 2004, I told both of them that their writing had saved my life.

Before that, the survivor stories people had posted on the site made me feel like I could one day feel less broken myself. I recently heard about the Survivors' Voices project here in the UK so, for more information on that, www.oneinfour.org.uk.

In the US, Ensler started V-Day because so many women were telling her their stories after each performance of *TVM*, she figured she had to either *do* something to help more or stop performing.

She's a great example of how we can expand our Circle of Influence **(23/12)**.

29/6 – Mariska Hargitay's Joyful Heart Foundation

Hargitay set up the Joyful Heart Foundation (www.joyfulheartfoundation.org) in response to fan mail. Hargitay's role as Lieutenant Olivia Benson on *Law & Order: Special Victims Unit* meant, like Ensler **(28/6)**, she heard stories of surviving rape and abuse.

Based in Hawaii as well as LA and NYC, Joyful Heart connects male and female survivors with their capacity for joy as well as offering support in seeking justice.

Hargitay founded Joyful Heart to make a difference. Since 2004, at time of writing, they have raised $28million and put more than 15,000 survivors through their healing programmes.

30/6 – Christiane Sanderson and shame

Sanderson is the author of several books about surviving childhood sexual abuse including *The Warrior Within* (One in Four, 2015). I did some training with her last year and this year and was especially taken by her talk of transformation. Trees of shame can become trees of growth. Just as Anodea Judith talks about harvesting our charge **(6/2)**, Sanderson says our shame leaves can fall off and become compost, helping us flourish.

Sanderson's approach emphasises the need to work on authentic **(3/7)** pride while working with shame in order to build resilience. Over the next several days **(1/7–4/7)**, I'll explain a bit more about different shame traps we can all fall into as well different types of pride which can help us heal.

You can find out more about Sanderson's work at www.christiane sanderson.co.uk.

July

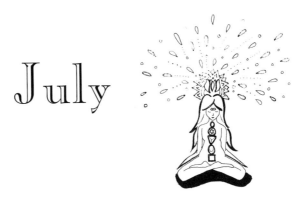

This month's tips include embracing our beach bodies, whatever our age, size and shape, the chakras, more mudras and yoga, more on shame and authentic pride.

1/7 – Releasing body shame

There's a whole industry devoted to spending millions of pounds encouraging us to feel ashamed of perfectly normal, natural things about ourselves. They hope that this shame will have us spend millions in an effort to correct the humanity out of ourselves. It kicks up a notch when ads start telling us how to get a 'bikini body' or 'summer body'. As if *any* body in a bikini or summer is somehow not a body.

Writing this, I know that some days, it's easy to recognise the cogs of industry behind our societal body shame. Other days, resistance is futile and we can catch ourselves feeling ashamed and worthless. Last summer, there was a huge backlash against an offensive 'beach body' ad campaign. Emblazoned across Tube platforms and buses, we recognised it as obnoxious and untrue. Unfortunately, when the messages are more surreptitious and, worse, inside our own heads, they're harder to defend against. But not impossible. We can be more mindful and get less sucked in.

The first time I saw the photos for this book – especially the ones with all my bellies - I was horrified. Reminding myself that I was able to *do* this photo shoot on Day 2 of my cycle **(28/2)** - in spite of my endometriosis and wearing thermals in a heatwave for better contrast in black and white - and that I'm strong, fit and healthy helped me be a bit kinder to myself about it.

What helps you appreciate your body for what you can *do* rather than fixating on how you look?

2/7 – Other types of shame

While body shame is something most women and, increasingly, men, have experienced, Christiane Sanderson talks about many other types of shame. These include:

- mind shame (whether to do with education or memory loss)

- abuse shame (where we internalise a sense of blame for what the perpetrator did)

- addiction shame (drugs, alcohol, sex, porn, gambling, spending, food or anything else)

- relationship shame (imagining everyone but us is normal)

- achievement shame (where our triumphs were downplayed so while we worked hard, we couldn't enjoy the results)

- sexual shame (with the added secrecy of having less of an idea of what other people consider normal)

- family shame and the intergenerational transmission of shame (where it can, like traumatic stress, be passed down. The plus side is that when we work on our own family shame, we can help heal the whole family system **(15/3)**)

- status shame (this can work in different directions depending on what the norms are in our social groups)

- gender shame (although, the transgender community are inspiring many of us by becoming more themselves)

- sense of self shame (where we feel inherently wrong)

- values shame (for example, a vegetarian surrounded by carnivores – or vice versa)

- culture shame (where we imagine others are better read, more musically and artistically astute) and

- aging shame.

We can simply scan the list to notice the ones that bring up the biggest charge **(6/2)** for us and prioritise working with those first.

3/7 – Authentic pride

Sanderson **(30/6)** says pride is essential when it comes to working with our shame. She differentiates between authentic and hubristic pride and gives the example of a toddler learning to walk. It isn't about being boastful or arrogant but acknowledging (even if just to ourselves) when we've done something well.

Increasing our sense of authentic pride has an added bonus: It's one of the positive emotions that has been proven to increase our DHEA levels **(2/12)**.

4/7 – Different types of pride

Sanderson **(30/6)** differentiates different types of pride we can all consciously develop to help us overcome our shame issues while developing more genuine confidence and self-esteem.

These types of pride include (and you may notice how this work can complement our shame work) pride in:

- communication

- achievement

- power and control

- relationships

- spirit

- what makes us unique

- social support

- skills

- comparison and

- growth.

Reading the list may spark an instant charge **(6/2)**. This can help us prioritise the most appropriate types of pride to work with first.

5/7 – How are your dreams trying to help you?

No matter *how* crazy our dreams seem, this Gestallt approach I learned from Martha Beck helps us look at each aspect as an aspect of ourselves. Even if it's someone we know in real life, it helps us identify the clues behind each element and character. It can be transformative. Too time consuming for all dreams (I typically remember at least three a night but only do this for the most vivid/disturbing), we can write the whole dream down.

Then we can take every element, describing it as if we *are* each element.

Then we can dialogue with it to find out how (in the dream) the crocodile/train/bathtub is trying to *help* us.

It can be especially challenging (and rewarding) with scary dreams. Yes, it requires some suspension of disbelief but can be a great way of communicating with our unconscious, often shifting what's felt stuck.

6/7 – Extreme self-care

No book on self-care would be complete without mentioning the Queen of Self-Care, Cheryl Richardson. The best-selling author of books including *The Art of Extreme Self-Care* and *The Unmistakable Touch of Grace* was booed by *Oprah Winfrey Show* audience members many, many years ago. She was a guest talking about the need for us to take better care of ourselves. This was before the 'put your own oxygen mask on first' analogy became the cliché it is today. Some mothers in Oprah's audience were outraged at the idea that their self-care could benefit their whole families.

Even though self-care is a more acceptable concept today, there are times when we're all challenged to put ourselves first. Just this week, a client said, 'So I need to become more selfish?' Recognising our triggers for feeling selfish (like we're somehow *wrong* to want whatever we want) can help us activate our favourite 'extreme' self-care practices.

7/7 – Irritation and pearls

Writing this, I am irritated, about a situation that's been going on for the best part of the year. In my opinion, it could have been nipped in the bud at the beginning. Yet I'm also aware that pearls form through oysters' irritation. Similarly, the lotus blossom **(19/12)** grows from the mud.

When we're in stinky, irritating situations, reminding ourselves of pearls and lotus blossoms can help us focus on how we'll take every opportunity to flourish.

This doesn't mean denying reality or 'thinking positive', but simply holding a longer view that beauty and value can come from what feels hideous in the present.

8/7 – Grit

Grit is where passion, persistence **(24/6)** and perseverance keep us focused on an important goal, according to University of Pennsylvania psychology professor, Angela Duckworth. The author of *Grit: The Power of Passion and Perseverance*, Duckworth encourages us to think less about talent and more about perseverance.

Reading about 'grit' helps me feel less shame **(27/6)** around some of the things I 'failed' first time around.

What 'singularly important goal' are you ready to apply grit to? **(17/11)**.

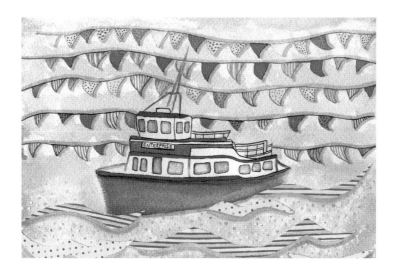

9/7 – Base chakra

When our base chakra (sometimes called root chakra) is in balance, we're grounded, secure, safe and well. We feel protected and have a balanced relationship to security and money.

If we're overactive in this area, we may focus too much on security and money. If underactive, we may feel unsafe and not have enough for our basic needs.

Grounding **(13/3)** is one of the best ways to balance our base chakra. Time barefoot in nature, even peeling potatoes or gardening. Reminding ourselves that our own energetic roots go deep and grow strong. Poses like Mountain, Warrior II **(20/2)** and mudras like Bhu **(29/10)** can also help.

Red **(14/5)** crystals, such as red jasper **(4/9)**, can be useful for working with our base chakras. While all come from the earth, the darker, heavier stones such as obsidian **(2/9)**, black tourmaline **(14/9)** and even rocks from the beach can be especially good for enhancing our sense of safety and protection.

I also find Louise Hay's affirmation, 'All is well. I am safe. Everything is working out for my highest good' helpful.

What helps you support your base chakra?

10/7 – Sacral chakra

When our sacral chakras are in balance, we're in the flow of life. Everything feels somehow easier. Creativity **(6/6)** comes easily and joyfully. We trust in life.

If our sacral chakras are overactive, we might become too spontaneous, failing to plan or prepare. If underactive, we might feel stuck. We're less likely to trust in life (or in anyone, including ourselves) and our creativity can feel like it has deserted us. Yoga poses that can help balance our sacral chakra include Cat/Cow **(16/8)**, Bow **(21/2)**, Wheel **(15/11)** and Pigeon **(18/8)**.

Orange **(15/5)** crystals are often associated with the sacral chakra area

and issues. These include carnelian, orange calcite and banded agate **(7/9)**.
What helps you balance your sacral chakra?

11/7 – Solar plexus chakra

When our solar plexus is in balance, we're in our power. We can be true to
who we really are without fearing exile. For our ancestors, exile would have
meant death.

If overactive, we may be overly aggressive rather than simply assertive.
When underactive, we may betray ourselves in a million little ways by not
stepping into our power when others overstep. We might tell ourselves it
doesn't matter but routinely putting others' needs ahead of our own isn't
healthy.

Power Poses **(26/11)** can be brilliant here. Yoga poses that can help
include the Warrior variations **(20/2)**, Triangle **(1/2)**, Seated twist **(31/1)**,
Supine twists **(29/1)** and Goddess.

Yellow **(16/5)** crystals that can help include citrine **(1/9)**, amber and
tiger's eye **(16/9)**.

What helps you balance your solar plexus?

12/7 – More on the heart chakra

This was introduced earlier **(25/1)**. You may notice that you feel differently
having, maybe, been working with it for a few months now? Does it feel
safer for you to open your heart centre more? Maybe you've learned to not
keep it too open?

Yoga poses that can help balance our heart chakras include Triangle **(1/2)**,
Warrior II **((20/2)** – keeping that strong, balanced grounding can make it

feel safer to open our hearts), Camel **(27/7)**, Cow faced pose **(26/7)**, Fish and Restorative Fish **(11/2)**.

Pink **(18/5)** crystals such as rose quartz **(30/8)**, pink tourmaline and green **(17/5)** ones such as jade, green calcite, amazonite **(13/9)**, aventurine **(9/9)** and pink *and* green ones like unikite **(8/9)** can help when we're working with heart chakra issues.

What supports your heart chakra?

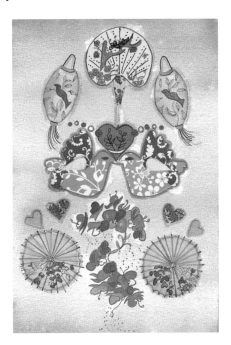

13/7 – Throat chakra

When our throat chakras are balanced, we speak (write, and even talk to ourselves) clearly, compassionately, truthfully and articulately. Giraffe In and Out **(17/2)**.

If overactive, we might be too 'honest' or simply talk too much. We might interrupt others - I am blushing writing this as I'm prone to this when out of balance.

When underactive, our expression is blocked. We bite our tongues and suppress our words. We might cry with frustration, unable to articulate our anger or hurt. Or we might simply stop bothering trying to express ourselves.

Chanting **(22/1)** can help with throat chakra issues. Neck rolls, Shoulder stand **(2/5)** and Fish **(11/2)** can also help.

Blue **(19/5)**, especially pale blue crystals such as blue lace agate **(5/9)**, blue calcite **(12/9)**, turquoise and sodalite can also support the throat chakra.

What helps you balance your throat chakra?

14/7 – Third eye chakra

When our third eye chakras are in balance, we trust our inner wisdom and guidance **(23/8)**, we're on friendly terms with our dreams **(5/7)** and we understand things easily. We also know how to turn our daydreams into goals and achievements.

If overactive, our dreams may become nightmares and we can struggle to make sense of what our intuition is almost bombarding us with. If underactive, we might find it hard to understand things and wonder if we even *have* dreams.

Yoga nidra **(9/3)**, body scans **(4/4)** and other guided visualisation meditations can all help balance third eye chakra issues.

Purple **(20/5)** crystals such as amethyst **(29/8)** and fluorite **(6/9)** can help, too.

What helps you keep your third eye chakra balanced?

15/7 – Crown chakra

When our crown chakras are balanced, we're in touch with the Divine (God, Goddess, the Universe, Nature, and our own Miraculous Self). Our every move and even thought feels guided.

If overactive, we may have spiritual crises and if underactive, we may forget we're all connected to this collective wisdom and grace.

Yoga poses that can help include Headstand, Hare **(28/7)** and Tree **(16/11** – especially when we open our arms above and imagine ourselves drawing down that healing sun energy into our whole energy field).

White **(29/7)** and gold **(30/7)** crystals such as snowy quartz and iron pyrite can help us work with crown chakra issues.

What helps you balance your crown chakra?

16/7 – More on the chakras

There has been an enormous amount written about the chakras. As an introduction, you might enjoy Sonia Choquette's *Balancing Your Chakras* and Anodea Judith's *Wheels of Life* and *Chakra Yoga*. Noticing which chakra we feel a lot of charge **(6/2)** around can be a wonderful way to work with them.

While people typically talk about balance and imbalance, as with any kind of 'balance' (such as the elusive 'work/life balance'), we're human. Any level of balance is typically temporary. By recognising the chakras we typically lose our balance around, we can kindly and compassionately take extra care of ourselves when we're in situations that add pressure.

None of this is about pathologising ourselves. Instead, we can use the ancient chakra system as a guide to help us find more harmony and balance with in our bodies, energy systems and lives.

17/7 – Chanting the chakras

This can enable us to tune into how we're feeling in any given moment. As with all chanting, our voices can indicate how our throat chakras are doing. Sometimes, I'm loud and clear, others, shy and almost ashamed.

All chanting helps elongate the exhalation **(9/1)**. The sounds are Lam (base **(9/7)**), Vam (sacral **(10/7)**), Ram (solar plexus **(11/7)**), Yam (heart **(12/7)**), Hum (throat **(13/7)**), Om (third eye **(14/7)**) and Ng (crown **(15/7)**).

To chant the chakras, do around 18 rounds of Lam, Vam, Ram, Yam, Hum, Om, Ng and as you notice how each vibrates in your system, notice which you may want to pay closer attention to.

Finish with three long ones, for example Yam, Yam, Yam.

Which chakra are you most drawn to working with today?

18/7 – Blowing bubbles

Yes, these are meant for small children. But bubbles can help us at any age. Apart from being beautiful when they catch the sunlight, blowing bubbles, like chanting **(22/1)** and singing **(2/3)**, naturally elongates the exhalation **(9/1)**, helping to calm our systems. They can be used indoors - carefully around food and electrical appliances - for space clearing as well as outside. Naturally uplifting, blowing bubbles can also help us connect with our inner child **(22/5)**. If we start out blowing them when we're feeling stressed out about something, we can imagine our stresses inside the bubbles, being carried away and recycled for the benefit of the planet. If that feels too gentle, we can imagine releasing each stress as we pop each bubble.

19/7 – Power talking

Amy Cuddy **(26/11)** points out that we can empower ourselves by the way we talk and deal with things as well as through our posture.

When we catch ourselves tripping over our words, talking quickly as if we don't think we're worthy of taking up space in the conversation, as well as working with our throat chakra **(13/7)**, we can simply slow down. Talking more slowly, like standing more expansively, helps us both feel and come across as more confident.

Similarly, when we respond instantly to emails, texts or other demands on our time, we may be being efficient or, if we're being too quick, we may be being reactive. We can notice whether we might be better off sleeping on something before responding, knowing that we don't have to march to the beat of someone else's drum.

20/7 – Open palmed mudra
To benefit from this simple mudra, rest the hands on the knees, palms facing up and open.

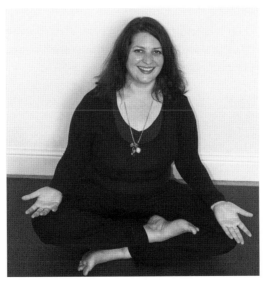

Some mornings, this is delightful and I can feel my hands tingling as I am actively open to guidance **(23/8)** for the day ahead. Other mornings, maybe I'm more stressed and wary and I find the fingers curling in protectively. I don't want to be so open.

It's another tool to aid mindfulness and adjust our approaches accordingly. Sometimes, we can deliberately open our palms (and hearts) more than feels comfortable and other times, we can honour that we don't *want* to be so open.

21/7 – Taking ownership of our devices

Studies show that the light from our phones and other devices can negatively impact our sleep quality, even contributing to insomnia. Still, sometimes, we simply want our phones *in* our bedrooms. I like my phone. It helps me be more extraverted from the comfort of my pjs. Yet, I notice that when I turn mine off a couple of hours before I intend to sleep and don't switch it back on again until after my morning meditation and yoga (nearest and dearest have the landline number for emergencies), my concentration *is* better. I feel more rested.

We all need to do what's best for ourselves. How do you feel when you imagine being less available to other people and more in tune with your own needs? (See also Digital Detoxes **(18/9)**.)

22/7 – Turning anxiety into excitement

There's an old coaching story about Bruce Springsteen and Carly Simon describing how they felt before going onstage. Bruce described heart racing, adrenaline and excitement, while Carly talked about anxiety and dread. Bruce was naturally turning his energy into excitement and even now – I am hearing from friends that his recent UK concert was the best performance they'd ever seen - delighting fans across the world. Carly temporarily gave into her stage fright.

Research backs up common sense. Allison Wood Brooks' paper, *Get Excited: Reappraising pre-performance anxiety as excitement* (2014, *Journal of Experimental Psychology*) encourages us.

It's far easier to reframe our anxiety as excitement than it is to instruct our whole system to 'calm down'. These words rarely work at the best of times **(29/2)**.

We can befriend our charge **(6/2)** when the adrenaline is pumping and even be more *open* to the idea of it being excitement rather than anxiety.

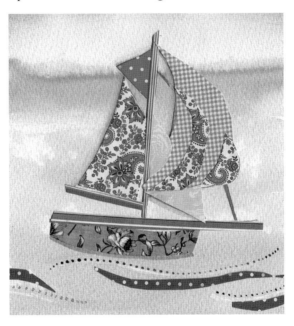

23/7 – Steeple Mudra

When it's inappropriate to take a Power Pose, we can benefit from Steeple Mudra. Amy Cuddy **(26/11)** writes about how world leaders often seem to naturally take this pose, creating more space with their hands (fingertips of both hands touching to create a steeple effect with the hands).

We can do it in a meeting, in a waiting room or pretty much any time. In yogic terms, it's known as Hakini mudra and said to aid concentration.

24/7 – Everyone else looks so serene

I remember noticing this in a class soon after I started practicing yoga. Exhausted from the pose, I caught sight of my reflection and realised no one else would necessarily know how much I was struggling.

When I teach, I encourage students to pay more attention to their body's wisdom than anything I say (while still building strength, stamina and flexibility) as I'm aware we can all look OK when we may feel the opposite. I was reminded of this again recently, attending a class taught by the lovely Emma Turnbull **(3/5)**. As my whole focus went on attempting the new pose, my inner critic **(3/10)** told me I was like a dancing dinosaur. When we released it, there was a collective sigh of relief and I was reminded that in yoga, as well as in life, we have no idea what's actually going on for other people.

I remember a line in Marian Keyes' *Rachel's Holiday* (Penguin, 1997) about how she was judging her insides against other people's outsides (what they presented to the world).

25/7 – Plough

Plough can aid digestion, alleviate stress, headaches and backaches.

- ✓ From Shoulder Stand **(2/5)**, simply bring the toes to the floor behind you, pausing for a few complete breaths, noticing how this feels.

- ✓ From lying on the mat, bring the arms alongside the body, bend the knees and gently lift the legs so the soles of the feet are facing the ceiling. Grounding through the arms, allow the knees to come towards you so the buttocks and hips lift.

- ✓ As you roll more onto the shoulders, move the hands to the lower back. Straighten the legs as they come towards the back of the head.

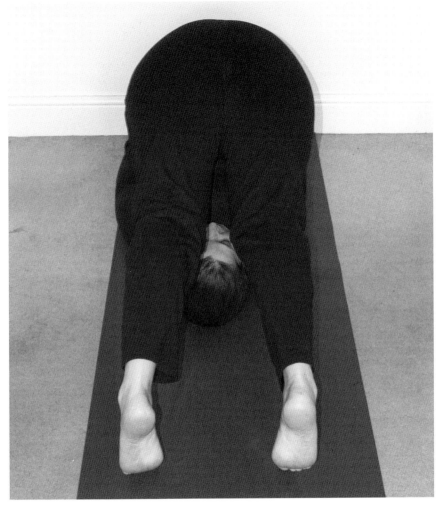

✓ Place the hands back down to the ground, bringing the toes as close to the floor as feels good. Keep the hips lifted by grounding through the arms.

✓ If the toes don't reach the ground, you can continue supporting the back with the hands. Notice the breath and, if comfortable to do so, aim to hold for five complete breaths. If you're holding any tension in the tongue or throat, you might release that.

Avoid if pregnant or you have any neck issues or untreated high blood pressure.

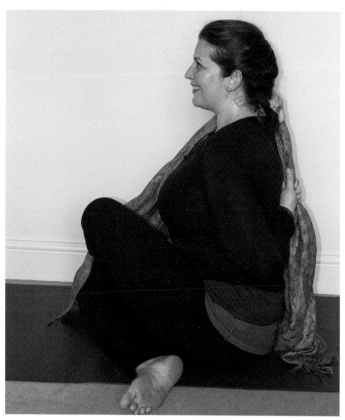

26/7 – Cow faced

A great stretch for the hips, thighs, shoulders and triceps, it can be helpful for some shoulder injuries while one to avoid for many. Notice how you feel looking at the picture, imagining going into it.

- ✓ From a cross legged seated position, stack the right leg so the calf comes over the left thigh. Check that you're balanced evenly on the sit bones.

- ✓ Put a strap (or scarf or belt) over the right shoulder. Take the right hand back, bend at the elbow, reaching it up between the shoulder blades and drawing it up to wherever feels best along the strap.

- ✓ Raise the left hand up and bend it behind the neck, drawing it down along the strap as far as it feels comfortable or until the fingertips can clasp together. You may not need the strap.

✓ Keep the spine straight, heart open and weight balanced on both sit bones. Notice your breath and, if comfortable, hold for five complete breaths.

If you don't want to do this as the hip stretch, too, it can be done from standing or sitting cross legged, just opening the heart centre and shoulders.

27/7 – Camel pose

✓ From a high kneeling position, tuck the toes under (unless you want a deeper back bend) and take the hands to the lower back/sacrum.

✓ Gently open the heart centre as you tilt the chin and head and lean backwards.

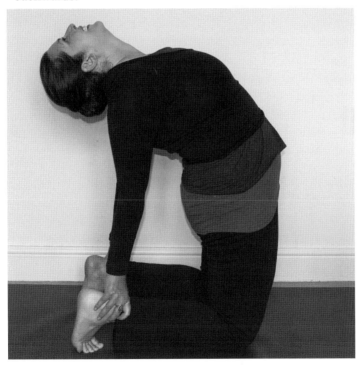

- ✓ This may be enough of a backbend for you or, if you want to go further, take the hands to rest on the ankles, keeping balanced, and reach the head towards the feet as you continue to open the heart centre upwards.

- ✓ Notice what's happening with the breath. As well as aiming to continue with your longer exhalation **(9/1)** and lower abdominal breath, Camel can be great for training the breath to the back of the lungs encouraging full thoracic breathing.

- ✓ If it feels good, stay for five complete breaths.

Camel can help bring us new perspectives as well as offering the mood boosting benefits of backbends.

28/7 – Hare pose

- ✓ Kneeling down, clasp the hands behind the lower back and gently fold forwards until the crown of the head rests on the mat. This used to hurt my head but it feels beneficial now. If your head is sore, you can add padding like a blanket or consciously put less weight onto the crown by putting the hands next to the head, taking some of that weight.

- ✓ If not, your hands may still be clasped behind your back, reaching up behind you to stretch the shoulders. Or they may be reaching back alongside your lower legs or reaching forwards, allegedly resembling the ears of a hare. Notice the breath, especially with the lungs, maybe, feeling quite compressed. Aim to stay for five to ten complete breaths if that feels good.

- ✓ Pause before coming up by resting the forehead on the hands for a few complete breaths.

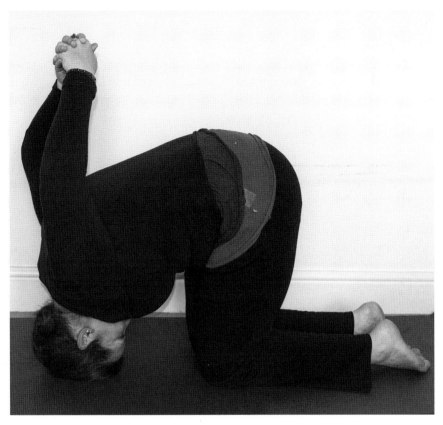

Hare is one of my favourite poses on mornings I am especially open to divine inspiration as it feels so crown focused. Some say it promotes healthy hair growth. Lisa Lister recommends it for Ovulation **(6/3)**.

29/7 – Gold

Gold is associated with the sun, prosperity, abundance, insight and the crown chakra **(15/7)** so can help us access that higher wisdom.

Golden light is also used in a lot of space clearing visualisations including one of my favourites from ENLP **(2/1)**.

30/7 – White

Associated with peace, healing, purification, protection and the moon, white is also linked with the crown chakra **(15/7)** and can help us tune into the Divine.

31/7 – Go wild

Whether we live in a city, town or countryside, there's always something we can benefit from by stepping out and noticing what we see. I've seen countless wild rabbits and even a deer along the local River Walk. London is filled with an abundance of parks and gardens. Inspiring as Cheryl Strayed's *Wild* journey was, we don't have to commit to anything so arduous to get some benefits.

'I always find walking in nature profoundly relaxing,' says Jini Reddy, author of *Wild Times* (Bradt, 2016). 'It gets me out of my head, helps me to shift any worries I'm carrying, awakens my senses, triggers creative bursts and makes me profoundly grateful for the beauty and mystery of the wild universe.'

Where are you reading this? How far would you have to venture to see woods? The sea? Fields? Mountains? Which kind of wildness is local enough and appeals? How do you feel in nature? Assuming it's good, how might you get out there more often?

August

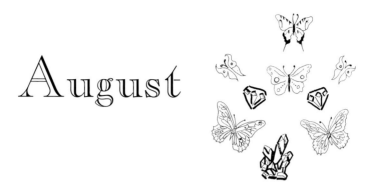

This month's tips include looking at what we've harvested from our efforts this year (and previous years) so far, forgiveness, working with crystals and EFT.

1/8 – Lughnasadh and harvest

This is a great time to take stock of how we're spending our time and energy. When we think about honouring our commitments, does our energy lift? Maybe we'd benefit from letting something go? It's also a time of reaping some of what we've sowed, while remaining patient for things that haven't yet come to fruition.

We can think back to when we started working with our charge **(6/2)**. We might notice how we've got better at befriending it, seeing how we feel in any given moment and asking ourselves how best to support ourselves.

As with everything, it's a practice. The more in tune we can become with what's going on in our bodies and minds, the better we can become at working with everything that arises, transforming our lives.

2/8 – International Forgiveness Day

Clichés abound regarding not forgiving being like taking poison and hoping someone else dies. Still, sometimes, we can really struggle to let go. Once we've done whatever it takes to ensure our safety, we can start reflecting on who we're most angry with. Often, it's with ourselves, for putting ourselves in a position that allowed us to be so hurt.

By going easy on ourselves, we can make more progress than by trying to be saints and turning other cheeks before we're ready.

If we can't forgive a particular person, maybe we can use today to become open to the possibility of forgiving them further down the line – again, while ensuring we're safe ourselves. Forgiveness is not about giving others carte blanche to hurt us again **(9/6)**. Maybe we're the ones who've behaved badly (we're all human). What might we do to make amends?

Even if, for today, we only manage to forgive ourselves a little, it's a step in the right direction.

3/8 – Gabrielle Bernstein's mindfulness of thought

One of my favourite mindfulness of thought tools comes from Gabrielle Bernstein's *May Cause Miracles* (Hay House, 2013). Noticing an unfriendly thought then saying (mentally, if in public), 'I forgive myself for that attack thought'. If anxious, 'I forgive myself for that fearful projection'. If comparing ourselves negatively to others, 'I forgive myself for making someone else special'. If comparing ourselves smugly to others, 'I forgive myself for making myself special.'

Personally, I find this more practical than just noticing the kind of thought **(13/6)** as it brings me more closure.

On occasion, where someone's really irritated me, I might notice myself having an unfriendly thought, try forgiving myself for that attack thought but more resentment bubbles up. Rather than trying to be a saint, I sometimes allow myself to indulge in *another* mean thought or two. Then I *properly* release it and forgive myself.

Mindfulness isn't about judging ourselves harshly for our humanity. By embracing our shadow as much as we can, we're less likely to project it onto others. Ultimately, it brings more peace.

4/8 – How long are our telomeres?

These DNA segments **(25/4)** at the end of our chromosomes get shorter each time our cells divide. This impacts a whole host of conditions we associate with aging. While scientists don't yet know whether short telomeres are a sign or cause of aging*, the more we can do to help keep our telomeres long, the better.

Eating antioxidant rich foods, exercising, yoga, meditation and generally keeping stress down can help keep our telomeres longer.

5/8 – Byron Katie's life changing questions

These questions can help us be more mindful of our thoughts and relieve much of the pain we create when we believe certain thoughts to be true.

Byron Katie has written several books about what she calls *The Work*. At the heart of it are four questions which we can apply to any painful thought.

In a nutshell, this means asking ourselves i) if the thought is true, ii) if we can truly know that for sure, iii) noticing how we react and the consequences when we believe that thought and, most liberating, iv) asking ourselves who we might be if we didn't have that thought.

You can find out more about her books, The Work and other processes at www.thework.com

---

* In terms of the body breaking down rather than chronological aging. I consider the latter a gift as it indicates we've been blessed with more time on this beautiful planet than the alternative would allow.

6/8 – Remember that you're safe right now

Whatever you've been through, whatever you've survived, you're safe right now, as you read this book. If you're in danger right now, please get yourself to a safe place! Our brains, bless them, don't always remember this. We can easily be triggered and flooded, feeling as if we're reliving traumas we've long since survived.

As well as being mindful of our breath **(7/1)**, staying as grounded **(13/3)** as possible is one of the best ways to hand this.

Simply feeling our feet, on the ground, tensing and releasing the thighs **(15/8)** or even stamping our feet are some simple ways to ground.

Others include using grounding crystals **(22/8)**, yoga asanas like Warrior II **(20/2)** and power poses **(26/11)**. EFT **(8/8)** can also help.

What helps you most?

7/8 – Star in your own story

If you were looking at a film poster of your life story, would you have top billing? If not, *who* would be getting the biggest credits? Where would *your* name appear? Would you even be in the small print below? Sometimes, we forget to be the suns in our own lives. We find ourselves orbiting others to such an extent, we forget ourselves and our own needs.

What would help you strengthen your gravitational pull so you get your attention back on your life and what *you* need and want?

You might also want to think about your nearest and dearest. How big would their names appear on their own film posters? Where would yours appear in relation?

Who do you know who has a good balance of being the star of their own life story while also having time for others?

8/8 – Introducing Emotional Freedom Techniques (EFT)

EFT (emotional freedom technique) is sometimes known as 'tapping'. It can be a great way of honouring our feelings, no matter how messy and complicated they feel. As an added bonus, we release blocked energy by tapping around some of the body's acupressure points.

When toddlers hurt, they cry, let it all out and generally recover very quickly. As we get older, we suppress things. By working with the meridians

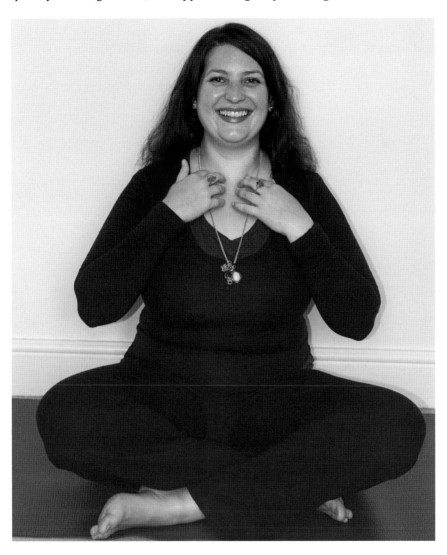

(the energy grids through the body that Chinese medicine works with), EFT can help us unblock that energy. We might laugh, cry or shake and it leaves us free from stuck emotions and even physical symptoms.

The next few days **(9/8-12/8)** introduce some simple tapping processes and tips on what to say.

9/8 – EFT Subjective Units of Stress (SUDS) scale

Sometimes, we can unblock emotions so quickly, we get bored or even forget why we started tapping. It's useful to grade our intensity of discomfort (or anguish) before we begin so we can measure it going up and down. On a scale of 0-10, how intense is the charge **(6/2)** around the situation? By being honest with how badly we're feeling with our situation, we can start shifting things.

Rating it also helps us access that wiser Self **(10/1)** that, even when in emotional or physical pain, can observe what's going on. We remember we're more than our issue.

It may just take one round (rare), a few, or several. Ideally, we want to take it down to a 0 but even reducing the intensity and going back to tap on it later can be better than nothing.

10/8 – The EFT Shortcut

Although there are more points to tap on, this Shortcut is appropriate for many issues. Starting with what's known as the Karate Chop point (edge of the hand), repeat the Set Up Statement **(11/8)** three times.

Moving to the inner eyebrow, tap there for the next sentence, moving to the outside of the eye for the next, under the eye, under the nose, the chin, the collarbone, under the arm (imagine the side of your, or a friend's, underarm at bra level) and then the top of the head.

Pause to take a deep breath, exhale fully and notice how you feel. Has your number changed? Initially, as we're really identifying with how badly we feel, it may go up – no need to be alarmed. When you have a new number (or the same), start again at the inner eyebrow.

We can tap on one side of the body or both sides at the same time – experiment with whatever feels best for you.

11/8 – EFT set up statement

There are lots of variations as some really struggle with this but the traditional set up statement is, 'Even though … , I deeply and completely love and accept myself.'

The … bit is the part that changes depending on what we're tapping about.

It might be, 'Even though *I'm terrified I'm going to lose my job/I'll never get over ____ /they can't diagnose this endless pain/I'm the worst parent on the planet/I keep overspending/I just can't handle this/whatever springs to mind for you.*'

The 'I deeply and completely love and accept myself' part is no picnic. I used to cry (no problem – tears help release that stress and blocked energy) myself and have seen countless clients cry or struggle with it. We can be kind to ourselves and if *too* painful, adapt it to something like, 'I'm OK.' This statement, even before we believe it, is self-soothing, calming the amygdala, letting ourselves know that even if nothing changes, we *are* OK.

12/8 – What to say as you tap other points

We don't need to add stress by worrying about what to say at each point. There's no right or wrong thing. We're simply voicing our feelings. Whatever we say is just right.

If, for example, you're overspending, it might be statements like, 'I'm overdrawn!', 'It's like I have no self-control', 'They'll have to give me a pauper's burial', 'Do they still *do* pauper's burials? Maybe they'll just leave me unburied!' – the more melodramatic the better at this stage. We're honouring that terrified part of ourselves by giving it a void while soothing it by tapping the meridian points.

Check in with yourself after each round and you'll find the phrases change as you feel better about it. There's no need to force or rush anything. When you've got all the fear out of your system, you'll naturally come up with reframes such as, 'I'm learning to take better care of my finances,' 'I'm open to abundance,' or whatever resonates with you.

We don't want to start with the affirmation type positives as we need to tap on what we're actually feeling. This is what frees us up to access our resources and make practical changes once we've tapped on it.

13/8 – Happy International Left-handers' Day!

Whichever side is dominant for you, why not celebrate difference today by experimenting with your other hand. Some people like writing from their unconscious selves with their non-dominant hand, gaining insights that their usual way of doing things might not be open to.

We can also take this chance to balance both sides of the brain with some Alternative Nostril Breathing **(7/4).**

In terms of behavioural patterning, even wearing a watch or activity tracker on the other wrist can bring additional new possibilities into our days.

How might you open up to a new way of doing something today?

152

14/8 – Trauma and movement

Peter Levine's ground-breaking work around trauma, *Waking the Tiger: Healing Trauma* (North Atlantic Books, 1997) helps us recognise that our responses are actually completely normal and appropriate.

The impala runs from the lion, plays dead then shakes it off before getting on with its day. Even if there was no lion, the impala doesn't appear to judge itself for overreacting. Those instincts (hopefully) keep it safe. We humans second guess ourselves for having been triggered. By being kinder to ourselves and understanding what's happening physiologically we can feel better faster. Our fight/flight/freeze response was triggered and we can move that energy through us by giving voice to our bodies **(3/4)**.

By noticing the physical sensations and honouring them, we can befriend our bodies. This is better than beating ourselves up for having reacted to something scary enough to trigger us, keeping the HPA-Axis flooding the system with adrenaline.

15/8 – Tensing and releasing the thighs

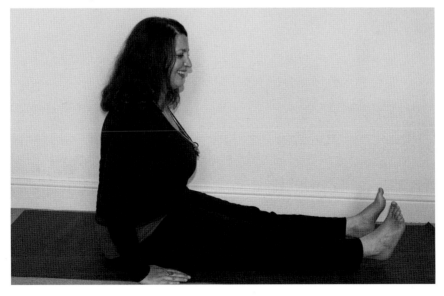

Another tool I learned from my yoga therapy training, based on Babette Rothschild's work, is simply inhaling as we tense our thigh muscles and exhaling as we release.

Often, we're triggered in situations where we can't immediately get it out of our systems by running (flight) or fighting **(3/4)**. Rather than getting stuck with the stress hormones flooding the body, we can tune into our breath as we tense and release.

We can be in a meeting and, if there's enough room, do this under the desk. If on a train or in a smaller space, we can tense and release the calf muscles. It's not as effective as the thighs (which have larger muscles) but a great way to get us into the present moment and remember that we are safe.

16/8 – Cat/Cow

Cat/Cow offers a gentle spinal and abdominal stretch. It's especially useful for becoming more mindful of the breath. Some days, it's easier than others

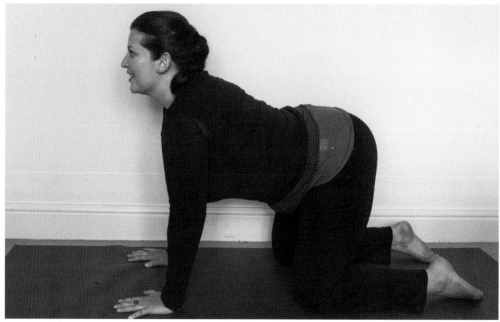

to co-ordinate the inhale as you look up, the exhale coming down. It's completely natural for minds to wander and we can simply choose to bring our focus back to inhaling up and exhaling down.

Because the movement's so simple, it's got enough going on to aid mindfulness. And it's not so complex that the idea of adding breath co-ordination makes you want to give up on yoga altogether.

Perfect for beginners, Cat/Cow pose is a helpful reminder to bring our awareness back to the body and the breath. This can be beneficial at any stage of yoga practice.

- ✓ Come to a tabletop position with your knees hip distance apart, hands either directly under your shoulders or slightly in front – experiment with what feels best for *your* body.
- ✓ Inhale as you lift the chin and head, looking up, then exhale as you round the spine and draw the chin towards the chest.
- ✓ Keep the moo-vement in time with the breath so the breath guides every move. For added calm, aim to breathe as if from the belly and have a slightly longer exhalation **(9/1)**.

17/8 – Cat/Cow variations

If kneeling is uncomfortable, ignoring your body's signals is not going to help you deepen your mind body connection. Instead, you may want to try a variation of the pose from standing or sitting. There are always options for modifying poses to be friendlier to *your* body.

- ✓ From standing, start with the feet hip distance apart. Bend the knees a little and rest the elbows on the thighs. You can make the stretch as deep as you want maybe bending the knees more. Inhale and look up, then straighten the legs as you exhale, bringing the head back down. Work with movement that feels good for you.
- ✓ From sitting in any comfortable position, inhale, lifting the head and neck back and exhale, rounding the spine and drawing the chin to the chest.

18/8 – Pigeon

With what we now understand about the fascia (that thin membrane that covers our entire bodies just below the skin) holding emotional memory, it makes sense that Pigeon pose is one of the best for releasing some of those blocked emotions. In this part of the world, our hips aren't as flexible as in parts where people routinely sit on the floor.

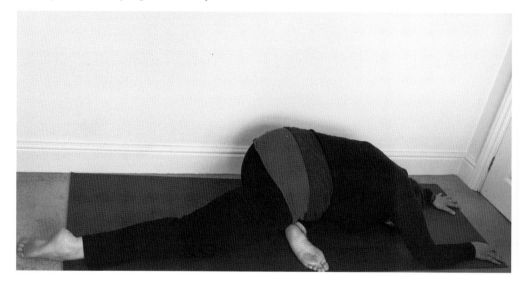

✓ Sitting on your mat, you can get into Pigeon by taking the right foot to the left side of the mat and the right knee at the right side. For a more gentle variation, point the toes towards the left hip. Keep the ankle muscles active.

✓ Lengthen the left leg back behind you by 'walking' the knee and toes backwards until you've dropped your pelvis down to feel a comfortable stretch. Enjoy the sense of grounding it can offer.

✓ Keep the left hip neutral. Fold forward, keeping the torso aligned, to whatever degree feels good for you.

✓ To come out, place your hands under the shoulders and push up. You can imagine yourself taking flight in the backbend version, pausing for a while there, if that feels good. Maybe even imagining yourself as a beauteous, open-hearted pigeon, taking flight in life. Expanding.

✓ In the forward fold version, it allows us to deepen our belly breath and elongate the exhalation even more **(9/1)**, cooling and calming the autonomic nervous system. In the backbend version, we can deepen our thoracic breathing **(3/3)**.

19/8 – Making time for our favourite people

We're interdependent mammals and often, when we're busy, we forget how nourishing our relationships can be.

Who haven't you seen enough of lately?

Who do you most want to reconnect with?

When was the last time you had so much fun you howled with laughter?

Building such times into our lives isn't just enjoyable – it sustains us. Y.C. Yang et al. back up research showing that strong social connections help us live longer, healthier lives.

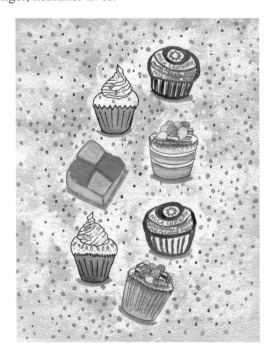

20/8 – Healing ball of light chakra yoga nidra

This is one of my favourite yoga nidras. I adapted it from one I learned from Shaura Hall (www.theyogologist.co.uk) and it's a simple one for you to do yourself.

- ✓ Starting by making yourself comfortable, lying on your back with your head, neck and spine aligned. Remember your sankalpa **(9/3)** or create a new one.
- ✓ Notice the sounds inside the room (even inside yourself) and outside the room, take yourself through the different parts of the body, rotating your awareness as you move from right hand thumb right around the body and head.
- ✓ Imagine a healing ball of shining light at your Crown centre **(15/7)**, getting bigger and brighter with each inhalation and smaller and dimmer with each exhalation.
- ✓ With each inhalation, let it heal that energy centre and all connected issues. Move this healing light from around your system. On the exhalations you choose move it from the Crown down to the Third Eye **(14/7)**. Then, Throat **(13/7)**, then to the right hand and arm. And then to the left arm before moving back to the Heart Centre **(25/1)**, Solar Plexus **(11/7)**, Sacral **(10/7)** and Base chakras **(9/7)**.
- ✓ Scan the whole body to return to any areas that could use some extra TLC. Remind yourself of your sankalpa before bringing your awareness back to the feel of the ground below you, air, temperature, sounds and so on.

Allow yourself to emerge feeling rested, alert, aware and relaxed.

21/8 – Self care

In psychosynthesis, the Self is the wise, observer part of ourselves **(10/1)**; it is known in other traditions as the Higher Self or Miraculous Self **(27/3)** or, even, soul.

While this whole book is about a year's worth of self-care ideas, today, we're focusing on Self care. When we tune in to this wise, compassionate inner guide, it can be quite transformative.

What does your Self, your *soul*, need today? How can you do more to nourish this precious part of yourself?

22/8 – Working with crystals

Crystal therapy was the first of the therapies I trained in. This training was my introduction to meditation and the catalyst for redesigning my whole life.

Drawn to crystals from my teens, I started intuitively using them for pain relief as I spent the best part of a year having a variety of hospital tests getting a chronic pain condition diagnosed. Since then, I've used them for almost everything. This includes space clearing, protection, manifestation, meditative focus, better sleep, grounding, travel and work.

Even Rainbow MagnifiCat has a crystal. She doesn't know it but any time she's out way beyond curfew and I get worried, I cleanse it to help keep me calm. Then, when she saunters on in, she rolls her eyes at me.

I use tumbled stones, shaped stones, rocks in their raw form and jewellery. The options are endless. These crystal focused days **(24/8-2/9, 4/9-9/9, 12/9-16/9 and 22/9-27/9)** might encourage you to play with them.

23/8 – Setting an intention and asking for guidance

Far more important than anything I or anyone else says about certain crystals being helpful for this, that and the other, is your *own* intuition.

The clearer we can be when we set our intentions **(4/1)**, the easier it is to tune into the best stones to use.

Settling, think about what you want the crystal to support you with. You could even create a sankalpa around it **(9/3)**.

Once you're clear, ask - Mother Goddess/Father God, Angels, Guides, Helpers, the Universe, your Miraculous Self, Grace; whatever feels most appropriate for you - for guidance and be quiet and still to listen to it before choosing your stone **(24/8)**.

24/8 – Choosing the stone

Once you've asked for guidance **(23/8)**, notice which stone/s you are drawn to. If you're at home or in private amongst your own crystals, you have more freedom. If you're out and choosing a stone to buy, remember to pay for it. Sometimes, the stone seems to communicate with a very clear, 'Me, me, meeeeeee!' and you just *know*.

Other times, we can see which ones our eye is drawn to or we can even hold a few or scan, using our non-dominant hand. This is associated with our unconscious wisdom. Some like to choose with shut eyes to better tune into this.

As long as we're clear about our intention, the right stone for each purpose will make itself known.

25/8 – Cleansing crystals

Once we've chosen stones, whether bringing them into our homes or choosing existing ones for a specific purpose, they need to be cleansed.

We can use incense, our breath, candle flame, moonlight, sunlight, burying it in the earth (although some find the earth reclaims them!), sound (ting tongs) or, my favourite, running water.

If you don't have access to a babbling brook (I would so love to have such access), water from a cold tap works fine. Some stones, like malachite, should be kept away from water.

Visualise any and all energies that aren't needed being released back into the earth, through the drain. They can be recycled for the benefit of the planet. I know how odd all of this can sound but we get a sense when stones need to be cleansed as well as when they have been.

Trust your intuition.

26/8 – Dedicating crystals

Once it's cleansed **(25/8)** ask that it be used only for the highest good of yourself and all concerned and dedicate it to be used for the highest love and light energies.

Then tune back into your intention and ask it to assist. Trust ideas that pop into your head about how best to proceed.

27/8 – Working with the stones

I believe they have their own vibrations and healing energy but even if you don't, stones and crystals can be great visual and kinaesthetic anchors. If you choose any for a specific purpose or goal, each time you see or feel it, you'll be reminded of this goal and more likely to take action.

There are so many other ways to work with stones **(22/8)**. I rarely sleep without one or two under my pillow, I have others around my home and workspace for space clearing and protection, I have some in my purse and bag. I even have stones in my drinking water **(22/3)**.

Sometimes, you might be guided to meditate with the stone, other times to maybe touch it to a painful part of your body or place it in a specific spot in your home. Experiment. Be playful and open to your guidance.

28/8 – Trusting your own intuition

There are many books about crystals **(22/8)** but the best guide is your own intuition. Think about it: You might read something specific about, say, rose quartz **(30/8)**. But how does it feel with *your* energy? Where in the world has the rose quartz rock you're holding come from? What energies has it been exposed to? How was it mined? How has it been treated? A rock may have a rawer energy than a pendant, shaped or tumbled stone. We don't need to be geologists to simply let go and trust our inner wisdom and guidance when working with stones.

Having said that, I know it can be daunting. I've included some associated meanings and uses I find helpful, having worked with crystals on a daily basis since 2001.

I hope you'll notice that the best possible crystal dictionary for you is one you may compile yourself from meditating with stones, dreaming and working with them in other ways. Trust yourself. And enjoy playing with the pretty stones.

29/8 – Amethyst

One of my favourites, this purple **(20/5)** stone comes in different shades, sometimes with white, too.

It is part of the quartz family. Often associated with the third eye chakra **(14/7)**, amethyst can help us tune into our inner wisdom. It can help us understand and work with our dreams **(5/7)**.

What springs to mind (colours, words, images, even sentences) when you meditate with an amethyst?

30/8 – Rose quartz

Also part of the quartz family, this pink **(18/5)** stone is associated with a gentle but strong kind of love and compassion. I always think of tough love.

Associated with the heart chakra **(25/1)**, it can help us connect to others and is often associated with romance. Most importantly, it can help us when working with self-care, overcoming self-loathing and learning to love and appreciate ourselves.

What springs to mind (colours, words, images, even sentences) when you meditate with a rose quartz?

31/8 – Clear quartz

If I could only choose one, I'd be sad. But I would choose this multitalented gem.

In sphere form, clear quartz can be used for scrying. It is often associated with clarity, protection and guidance.

Clear quartz is a very powerful stone. I imagine it almost like the Tower card in the Tarot. It can help us shift stuff but sometimes, something gentler can make it a smoother transition.

Shape matters **(18/9)**. A sphere, pendant or tumbled stone will have a different energy to a double terminated quartz wand. Experiment. Notice what you're guided towards.

What springs to mind (colours, words, images, even sentences) when you meditate with clear quartz?

September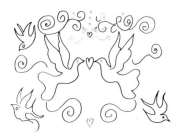

This month's tips include more on crystals, releasing blocked feelings and emotions safely, inner strength and peace building from the inside out.

1/9 – Citrine

Another member of the quartz family, citrine is yellow **(16/5)**, often with white. I see it as a little ray of sunshine, helping to boost moods, find joy and grace. It's sometimes associated with the solar plexus chakra **(11/7)** and can help us empower ourselves in a playful, fun way.

It is also sometimes associated with abundance and manifestation.

What springs to mind (colours, words, images, even sentences) when you meditate with citrine?

2/9 – Obsidian

This beautiful black stone is great for grounding, protection and absorbing energies and pain (so we need to cleanse, cleanse and cleanse).

It can be held during meditations to help us connect with the earth's grounding energies. As well as loving the rock obsidian stones I have, I keep a stunning obsidian sphere with my clear quartz one for balance and protection.

What springs to mind (colours, words, images, even sentences) when you meditate with obsidian?

3/9 – Back to school?

Whether you're heading back to school yourself or getting the kids ready for a new academic year, September offers a 'blank slate' energy offering new beginnings. Expansiveness. When we learn, we create new neural pathways and help our brains stay healthy and well.

What would you love to learn more about? Notice any limiting beliefs that may crop up ('If I were younger/had more money/whatever') and allow yourself to imagine yourself opening a door to new learning in your life right now.

It may be formal learning (a course of some kind) or you might decide to explore a subject or area that's piqued your interest.

4/9 – Red jasper

Red jasper has an earthy reddy orange colour and sometimes includes white. It is often associated with the base chakra **(9/7)** and can be brilliant for grounding, manifestation and protection.

During a particularly fragile-feeling winter, decades ago, I used to put some red jasper inside my glove for extra grounding and protection. A small stone in your bag or purse can be enough. Red jasper has such a warm and protective energy, I often use imaginary red jasper in my morning space setting meditations **(3/1)**.

What springs to mind (colours, words, images, even sentences) when you meditate with red jasper?

5/9 – Blue lace agate

This gentle pale blue stone has gentle stripes running through it. Like rose quartz **(30/8)**, blue lace agate can be great for encouraging self-care.

Blue lace agate is often associated with throat chakra issues **(13/7)** so can help us when we struggle to express ourselves.

It is also sometimes associated with angelic energy.

I sometimes combine, for example, the gentler blue lace agate energy with obsidian **(2/9)**, tourmaline **(14/9)** or hematite appreciating the heavier grounding energy as back up.

What springs to mind (colours, words, images, even sentences) when you meditate with blue lace agate?

6/9 – Fluorite

This beautiful crystal combines purple **(20/5)**, clear quartz and green. I think of the Suffragettes due to the colour combination as well as loving it for Earth, Link, Flow **(20/3)** meditations. It is sometimes associated with synthesis, bringing things together and integrating them for a greater whole. Due to its colours, fluorite is also sometimes associated with heart chakra **(25/1)** and third eye chakra **(14/7)** energies.

What springs to mind (colours, words, images, even sentences) when you meditate with fluorite?

7/9 – Banded agate

Part of the agate family, this shares blue lace agate's **(5/9)** gentle power. An especially pretty stone, it blends whites and pinks and browns and other colours.

Sometimes associated with integration and synthesis, it can offer gentle but powerful assistance in these areas.

What springs to mind (colours, words, images, even sentences) when you meditate with banded agate?

8/9 – Unikite

This blends a grassy green **(17/5)** with pink **(18/5)** so is doubly associated with the heart chakra **(25/1)**.

It can bring strength when dealing with loss, heartbreak and grief, reminding us that we are whole no matter what. Unikite offers gentle empowerment when even the smallest things feel too challenging.

What springs to mind (colours, words, images, even sentences) when you meditate with unikite?

9/9 – Aventurine

This stunning green **(17/5)** stone can be healing, regenerative and restful. It is also sometimes associated with abundance and manifestation.

It makes me think of adventure and newness. Also associated with the heart chakra **(25/1)**, it has a buoyant, invincible energy that can help us remember to let our hearts lead us sometimes.

What springs to mind (colours, words, images, even sentences) when you meditate with aventurine?

10/9 – World Suicide Prevention Day

When we feel so down there feels like only one way out, the thought of ending things can be a relief. I'm grateful, looking back, that my early teenage attempt failed and put me off trying again. No matter how bad things felt afterwards, there was a part of me that remembered my gratitude when it hadn't worked or done any permanent damage.

None of our feelings are permanent. Joy, pain, it's all temporary. Recognising that suicidal thoughts can just be a way of blowing off steam means we can indulge them without acting on them. Like married people who sometimes fantasise about divorce.

If your suicidal feelings feel more serious, please talk to someone: a loved one, your GP, the Samaritans or a therapist.

It *will* pass. We can overcome whatever we're dealing with. There is more to you than whatever it might be. Seeking help takes courage and can be scary but we can turn our lives around.

www.samaritans.org and see www.iasp.info/wspd for more information on the prevention day.

11/9 – Wisdom

Another Universal Strength **(31/5)**, Wisdom is considered to be a higher form of intelligence. It helps us put our own and others' wellbeing ahead of momentary pleasures. The Children's Fire **(5/6)** epitomises wisdom for me. Native American elders would not be swept up by short term gain to bankrupt their children's futures.

Overplayed, we might take life too seriously and not have any room for spontaneity. Underplayed, we may act foolishly.

How might you hone your wisdom today?

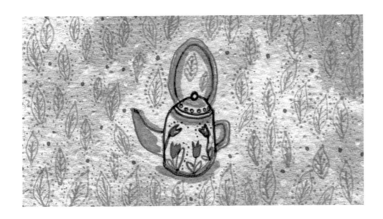

12/9 – Blue calcite

This soothing, milky blue stone is associated with the throat chakra **(13/7)**. Its gentle, calming energies can be useful before or during presentations.

I sometimes choose blue calcite for under my pillow when I want to encourage especially sweet dreams.

What springs to mind (colours, words, images, even sentences) when you meditate with blue calcite?

13/9 – Amazonite

This glorious, lush green **(17/5)** stone is often linked with the heart chakra **(25/1)**. I associate it with an even bolder energy than aventurine **(9/9)** and it can be great for giving us the courage to live more whole-heartedly.

What springs to mind (colours, words, images, even sentences) when you meditate with amazonite?

14/9 – Black tourmaline

This beautiful black stone has grains like a Flake chocolate, although it's usually wider. And not edible!

I appreciate its grounding, protective energy as an aid for sleep. It can help us connect with the earth's nourishing energy while helping us release what we no longer need. I regularly incorporate imaginary tourmaline into my meditations for extra grounding and protection.

What springs to mind (colours, words, images, even sentences) when you meditate with tourmaline?

15/9 – Labradorite

This stunning stone is easily recognised by its chatoyancy (iridescent shimmering surface) and looks greeny, greyey, blue depending on the stone and light.

Protective and grounding, labradorite is also great for when we're moving into a more expansive way of being. When we're playing bigger and maybe feeling unsafe while also ready to flourish. Labradorite can help us honour these sometimes conflicting feelings and integrate them.

What springs to mind (colours, words, images, even sentences) when you meditate with labradorite?

16/9 – Tiger's eye

Available in gold/yellow and blue, tiger's eye is also known for its chatoyancy **(15/9)**.

While yellow or gold tiger's eye is associated with the solar plexus chakra **(11/7)** and blue the throat **(13/7)**, both can help us connect with our personal power. Tiger's eye can support us in expressing ourselves and, when necessary, roaring to make ourselves heard.

What springs to mind (colours, words, images, even sentences) when you meditate with tiger's eye?

17/9 – Eye exercises

'Reading and working on screen is like running for our eyes, rather than walking or sitting,' says Francesca Marchetti, an ocular specialist on the impact of digital technology (www.digitaleye-d.co.uk). Francesca recommends pausing after every 20 minutes of screen time. By giving our eyes a 20 second break (looking at something 20 feet away), we can reduce digital eye strain and the headaches and blurred vision associated with them. She also suggests blinking 20 times. Each time I do this, it feels like my eyes have benefitted *and* it makes me laugh – extra boost.

18/9 – Digital detox

Much as I adore my smartphone, tablet and laptop, I know that it's important to remember it's up to *me* how much I use them. I don't enjoy being sucked down the digital rabbit hole and over doing things. Research commissioned on behalf of Bausch + Lomb ULTRA, looking at 1000 adults aged between 20 and 60 found that 58.8% of women and 39.4% of men use their phones as comfort blankets.

How you feel as you read the words 'digital detox'? Do you feel anxious at the idea of 24 hours (or even 12, 8, 4 or even 1 hour – this is for your benefit. Do what's best for you and your lifestyle) without your devices? Maybe the very idea feels like freedom?

By having regular 'digital detoxes', we not only help our eyes rest, we remind ourselves that they're a relatively recent invention. We *are* whole without them. We can choose when to switch them off and on **(21/7)**.

19/9 – Smoky quartz

This looks similar to clear quartz **(31/8)** but has a smoky look to it. Smoky quartz helps me during those times when I want support in managing life's uncertainties and complexities.

Sometimes, much as I might crave the clarity and simplicity of clear quartz, smoky quartz helps me stay with the reality.

What springs to mind (colours, words, images, even sentences) when you meditate with smoky quartz?

20/9 – Autumn Equinox approaching

Tomorrow, also known as Mabon, is a great time of year to ponder balance, as light and darkness are equal. We can also think about what we've harvested, what we're releasing and where we're heading.

It's a great time to take time to be grateful for all we have. We can honour our efforts in getting there, too. By noticing what no longer serves us, we let go in order to grow.

It's also a good time to be open to guidance around treading lightly, living as harmoniously with the earth as possible. What we release energetically can be transmuted to benefit the planet.

21/9 – International Day of Peace

The UN's International Day of Peace (http://www.un.org/en/events/peaceday) was created to imagine warring people setting differences aside for just one day. If they could do it for one day, the hope was that they'd build on it.

By bringing more peace to our own lives, we can better contribute to (yes, I'm still an idealist) world peace.

We can use the EFT **(8/8)** Personal Peace Procedure to help us, too. List everything you can think of that disturbs your peace and tap on it.

22/9 – Hematite

This heavy, silvery grey metal rock is fantastic for grounding and protection. It's another stone that can be great under the pillow, creating a safe enough feeling for sleep. I often mix its energies with something gentler like amethyst **(29/8)** or blue lace agate. Use whatever you're drawn to.

Like obsidian **(2/9)** and tourmaline **(14/9)**, hematite can help us handle what might feel like negative, toxic environments, not that we should stay in such situations, but helping us until we're able to leave.

It can absorb some of that negativity and we can keep cleansing it, visualising it being released from the stone and from our situation.

What springs to mind (colours, words, images, even sentences) when you meditate with hematite?

23/9 – Snowy quartz

This white stone has the strength of its quartz family and gentle, purifying qualities.

I like using this with hematite, obsidian **(2/9)** or tourmaline **(14/9)** as a way of bringing lightness. It can help us connect with our crown chakra **(15/7)** and to be open to guidance and wisdom.

What springs to mind (colours, words, images, even sentences) when you meditate with snowy quartz?

24/9 – Snowflake obsidian

This black stone with white spots naturally brings the optimism of, for example, snowy quartz to the gorgeous grounding of the obsidian **(2/9)**.

It can help us tap into a sense of optimism no matter how messy things have felt.

What springs to mind (colours, words, images, even sentences) when you meditate with snowflake obsidian?

25/9 – Shapes of crystals

As mentioned **(28/8)**, the shape influences the energy of each stone. Some shapes are softer, others more raw and jagged, some pointy, some spherical. Notice which shaped stones you're most drawn to. As well as using crystals, stones on a beach offer a range of shapes to play with. These ordinary rocks have grounding properties too.

26/9 – Crystals in jewellery

I never put on jewellery without thinking how I want it to help me feel **(22/8)**. I usually wear several pendants at the same time, earrings, rings and bracelets.

Over time, these pieces can anchor specific qualities for us. It offers a simple and effective way to remind ourselves each time we see them that we're aiming to bring more grace, peace, joy, adventure or whatever into our lives.

It also allows experimentation, adding different types of stones to our energy fields and noticing how they work in harmony (or not) with each other.

27/9 – Choosing crystals for others

Sometimes, when loved ones are going through something, as well as asking how we can help and sending Metta **(15/2)** we can ask for guidance when choosing a stone **(24/8)** to best support them. We can ask their Miraculous Self **(27/3)** for permission and guidance as well as tuning in and setting a clear intention.

Obviously, this is intention is for our loved one's highest good rather than us potentially thinking we know exactly what they need and possibly (probably) missing the bigger picture.

We can also choose stones to help us better support loved ones. For example, we might be feeling very anxious about a loved one's anxiety. By supporting ourselves with our *own* anxiety (and owning the fact that we *have* our own), we help them more.

The world is your lobster. We can choose crystals to help ourselves with absolutely anything.

28/9 – Releasing old energies into the sea

On a recent holiday to a Greek island, I had one of my best ever sea swims. Apart from being fun, it felt like it was washing away everything that's ever held me back. I did a spontaneous underwater Happy Dance.

Even when it's too cold to swim in the sea (I usually swim off Essex's 'sunshine coast'), we can choose a pebble or rock. Holding it in our right hand (associated with our more active side), we can ponder what we're ready to release - old dreams, energies, habits, whatever springs to mind. You know yourself best.

When you're ready, fling it as far into the sea as possible. Visualise yourself releasing all that you are ready to release. Know that the sea can take all that energy and transmute it for the benefit of the planet.

29/9 – Pre-menstrual

This autumnal, waning (lessening) lunaresque phase gets a bad rap. Falling oestrogen, progesterone and testosterone (assuming we didn't get pregnant) can leave us feeling withdrawn.

Lisa Lister **(28/2)** points out that what some might consider moodiness is actually our 'feminine super-powers' kicking in. We can tap into our intuition and yes, some might see us as irritable but it's actually a great time for assessing our lives. We can prune things back, make more time for ourselves and let go of what no longer works.

Our critical thinking capabilities are higher now and we can get organised and practically bulldoze any creative blocks.

30/9 – Flush it

Sometimes, the thoughts draining our energy, going round and round, can make us feel quite stuck. The more we think those thoughts, the more they get entrenched in our brains, having created new neural pathways. This kind of thought then becomes our default thinking.

One of my favourite, quick ways to break this spiral is to make a quick note of whatever's bugging me that I'm ready to release. I use biro on loo roll then flush it down the loo.

It can help us take our concerns more lightly as well as reminding ourselves that we are more than whatever thought pattern we feel stuck in.

October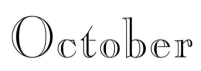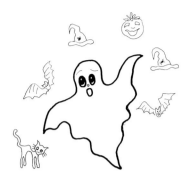

This month's tips include more ideas for releasing stuck energy, reaching out for support (and fun), lessons from self-harm, some NLP and more yoga.

1/10 – Writing a letter and burning it

The idea of closure is very appealing. Of course, real life rarely works that way. Instead, we can write a letter to that ex, boss, parent, friend, predator or whoever is taking up too much of our headspace rent-free.

This isn't about whoever we're writing to - we're not *sending* it. We're simply releasing some of that trapped energy. Just as tracking our somatic sensations and completing a physical action can help in trauma work **(14/8)**, expressing ourselves safely in this way can help us honour our feelings about whatever the issue is.

We can write until we've said everything we currently have to 'say' to the person. Then, most importantly, destroy the letter. We can shred it, rip it up, burn it (safely) and pause to notice how we feel.

Sometimes it just takes one letter, other times a whole series. Each one helps us release whatever we're ready to release at that time.

2/10 – Deciding what we want to actually express

Sometimes **1/10** is enough. Often, by freeing ourselves by (safely) saying the previously taboo, we realise we're actually ready to express some of it to the person. When this is the case, we might draft a letter or email – remembering to leave the address field blank - to send them or even note down key points for a phone call or conversation.

Again, by pausing to notice how we feel at different stages (even imagining talking to the person or hitting Send), we can better tune into the appropriate response.

We can even visualise the recipient reacting in the way we most hope for and edit our letter to help us make this outcome as likely as possible.

3/10 – Inner critic

I've been working on my own propensity to mentally rip myself to shreds for years. Knowing that no matter what's going on, self-flagellation triggers the stress response while soothing ourselves helps activate the parasympathetic branch **(9/1)** means I've continued to work with it.

While most people have heard of fight/flight, 'tend and befriend' is another helpful response. Shelly Taylor says many people, especially women, react to stress by ensuring those around them are OK. Soothing self-talk helps us help others as well as ourselves. It's still* very much a practice. Some days are easier than others and certain tasks mean my negative self-talk is more likely to be my default.

My mindfulness practices **(7/1)** at least help me notice this and my cat has been a superstar. I'd never want Rainbow MagnifiCat to be scared of anything I did. By talking soothingly to her no matter what's going on, I've become that much more soothing talking to myself.

Who might you imagine talking to more kindly? Dog? Cat? Toddler? We can also work with our Inner Critic subpersonality **(10/1 and 3/10)**.

---

* and this is my *work*.

4/10 – World Animal Day

Whether you have pets and regular contact with animals or not, how does the notion of World Animal Day feel? Totally uninteresting? Wistful, as you spend every day resisting a trip to your local animal shelter to adopt an animal in need?

Beyond pets, we can ponder spirit animals. In Elizabeth Gilbert's *Super Soul Sunday* special with Oprah, she talked about taking herself for a walk into the local wildlife on New Year's morning and being open to meeting her spirit animal for the year ahead.

We might lack her back doorstep wilderness but asking our inner guides **(25/2)** for a sign from the animal world can be illuminating. We can then meditate on (and even Google) our spirit animal and see what resonates for our own lives.

5/10 – Negative self-talk

Just as many of us of us have strong inner critics **(3/10)**, we often unconsciously put ourselves into trances with endless negativity.

'Oh, I'd be rubbish at that. I can't do anything. Sure, someone else might be able to learn quickly but not me. Just can't do anything.'

If anyone else were to say to us, 'Oh, you're rubbish. You can't do *anything*,' we would be outraged (at least, a teeny tiny part of ourselves would be), recognising the emotional abuse. Inside our own heads, though, we rarely challenge it. This is *not* about 'thinking positive' and beating ourselves up for being humans with a full and complex emotional spectrum.

Noticing the language we use with ourselves, as well as the tone - Compassionate? Harsh? - can lead to pretty radical changes in a gentle way.

6/10 – The three legs of NLP

In a nutshell, NLP comes down to:

- ✓ setting a well-formed outcome
- ✓ noticing the feedback we get from the world and
- ✓ adapting our approach accordingly so we're more likely to attain the result we're after.

The next few days **(7/10 - 9/10)** go into each element in more detail.

7/10 – Setting a well formed outcome

This is just another way of saying goal. It's important to make it positive (similar to a sankalpa **(9/3)**) as our conscious minds struggle to process a negative.

For example, when I quit smoking, I decided to focus on becoming a healthy, happy non-smoker rather than saying 'quit smoking'. Even though I quit in 2001, typing the latter still makes me want a cigarette now. Stating our goals as simply and positively as possible makes it easier to focus on what we *want*.

8/10 – Sensory acuity

Or, as Dr Phil might say, 'How's that working for you?' This is where we can measure the progress we're making towards our well-formed outcomes. Is what we're doing getting us closer, keeping us stuck or even moving us further away from what we ostensibly want?

There are all sorts of ways to pay attention. One radical seeming but effective method is to ask those who observe us (and want us to succeed) for feedback.

What do they spot that our blind spots conceal?

If not yet brave enough to be so vulnerable **(27/6)**, observing our own efforts - honestly and compassionately - can be transformative.

9/10 – Adapting our approach

We can set all the well-formed outcomes we want **(7/10)**. We can even be honest with ourselves about what's working and what's not **(8/10)**. But if we're not prepared to do something differently and to *keep* adapting our approach as necessary, nothing will actually change.

Sensory acuity **(8/10)** is like mindfulness, powerful and potentially transformative. Actually doing something different is the regulation element. The instant relief part of the puzzle. It can be challenging (especially when we've been in certain ruts for a long time - it takes effort to create those new neural pathways) but worth it.

What happens when you imagine applying these three simple steps **(16/10)** to any area of your life you're keen to improve?

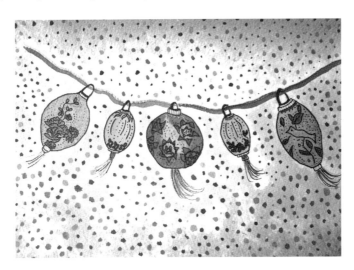

10/10 – Happy World Mental Health Day!

While much is being done to raise awareness of different conditions as well as reducing stigma, many people feel isolated and ashamed in ways we simply wouldn't about, for example, seeking treatment for a broken leg.

On this designated day (www.mentalhealth.org.uk/campaigns/world-mental-health-day), we can all do a mental MOT on ourselves.

What's working well? Where do we feel more fragile or wobbly? What triggers us?

What helps (when we give ourselves permission to listen to our inner wisdom)?

When we're well, we can look beyond ourselves and reach out to offer support (in a tentative, respectful way) to someone we see who may be struggling.

11/10 – Coming Out Day

'Be yourself,' say so many well-meaning people. But when we feel out of place, this can feel scary. Unlike race and gender, sexuality is often something people feel unable to be open about for fear of reprisal. Even now, homophobic and transphobic attacks are too commonplace.

Apart from sexuality, there are all sorts of things we can feel uneasy about 'coming out' around - from political allegiances to spiritual beliefs. Susan Cain's bestseller *Quiet* (Penguin, 2012) explores being introverted in a world where extraversion is admired. Teachers discuss children with introverted tendencies furtively with parents, as if a glitch to be fixed.

The more I see people expressing themselves (be it through living as the gender they feel, loving whoever they love, or even wearing whatever they feel like), the more my own heart sings. Being ourselves frees other people.

Is there an aspect of yourself you'd like to honour (even if only to yourself) today?

12/10 – Our bodies can help us connect

While Amy Cuddy's work **(26/11)** shows us how we can use our body language to feel more embodied and at ease in our own skin, we can also use our posture to boost our connections.

Relationship coach Elena Angel **(29/5)** recommends turning towards our loved ones, even if we naturally want to turn the other way or cross our arms in front of ourselves.

Being mindful **(24/3)** about our body language helps us think about how it might make someone else feel. We can also be more conscious about the signals we're sending our own brains. We can choose - if we want to - to nip things in the bud by staying open and loving with our whole selves.

13/10 – Goal setting

Without goals (or well-formed outcomes **7/10**), it's easy to bob through life moving further from what we want. This isn't about draining life's spontaneity by creating five or ten year plans (unless that's something you love to do).

What's important to you? What makes your heart sing? What sparks joy **(19/3)**?

Creating a vision board **(24/12)** can help us notice what energises us. Setting a sankalpa **(9/3)**, goal or well-formed outcome keeps it at the forefront of our minds while also allowing our unconscious minds to work their magic.

14/10 – Powerful goal setting

Along with the Logical Levels **(17/11)**, this is one of my favourite goal setting tools. I learned both during my NLP training.

POWER helps us remember:

P (positive) - we're stating our goal in the positive **(7/10).**

O (obstacles) - to ponder probable and potential obstacles before we even start so we can plan to put better supports in place for ourselves rather than getting blindsided and knocked off track later.

W (way forward) - to contemplate our next steps and milestones along the route from where we are to where we want to be.

E (ecology) - my favourite, this step reminds us to anticipate the effects of reaching our goal will have on our wider ecosystem. Loved ones, our team or organisation, community and even the planet. By anticipating the implications, we can reassess our goals and reassure those around us about concerns.

R (resources) - this is where we can start preparing to move full steam ahead, identifying all the resources we already have as well as those we can seek out. From books and training to people and even our own willpower.

15/10 – What stops you accessing all your resources?

We're often more resourceful than we give ourselves credit for.

Mindfulness **(24/3)** can still the mind enough to help us draw on the knowledge, wisdom and resources we already have.

Power posing **(26/11)** can help us feel brave enough to reach out to others for support.

When you think of times you haven't accessed all your resources, what stopped you?

Knowing this about yourself, how can you better support yourself in accessing all your resources in the future?

16/10 – World Food Day

We are so lucky to have access to so many delicious foods from around the world as well as local produce. At the same time, many of our foods lack the nutrients our ancestors got as we humans have affected the soil. Still, we can give thanks for the support and nourishment our food brings us.

Which foods nourish you the most? Which don't agree with you? Which taste delicious but don't offer any nutritional value? When we pay more attention to where our food comes from and the effects on our health and wellbeing, it's amazing how we feel less need to comfort eat.

We can also donate to local food banks and get involved with other charities (like www.fareshare.org.uk and www.foodcycle.org.uk) to help people struggling to provide nourishment for themselves and their families.

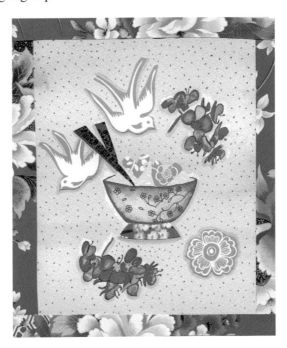

17/10 – Self-harm with food and other compulsions

We've all done something that didn't contribute to our self-care. Mine include tearing my hair out (from 11 to 34), drinking too much in my teens and twenties and failing to notice that all the 'muscle' I gained when I replaced smoking and alcohol with yoga, swimming and cycling was actually fat from comfort food.

While shame and self-loathing can be high with any unhealthy habit, beating ourselves up just triggers the amygdala **(23/5)**. This leaves us in need of *more* comfort through food, drugs, drink, self-harm, spending or gambling.

It's still (very much) a practice, but when I look behind my unhealthy habits to the need (for comfort, safety or whatever) behind it, I'm better able to find healthier ways of meeting those needs.

What helps *you*?

18/10 – Friendly finances

Our overspending and self-sabotage around earning can be another thing that gets in the way of self-care. Money means we can afford the things that boost our wellbeing (from therapy to a massage).

Even small savings can help us free ourselves from toxic work environments or living arrangements.

How do you feel about your current situation?

What would be a small, manageable step in terms of your financial self-care?

19/10 – How do you feel about your spending?

Kate Northrup, author of *Money: A Love Story* (Hay House, 2013), suggests doing an emotional inventory by looking at credit card and other statements and noticing which spending makes us smile and which makes us frown. Similar to Marie Kondo's clutter clearing method **(19/3)**, releasing everything that doesn't spark joy, Kate encourages us to tune into our feelings around spending.

As we look at bills (aka 'blessings already received') we get a sense of the kind of spending that, to us, *is* worth it. Which items make us beam? Which have we already forgotten? This makes it easier to eliminate silly spending without feeling deprived.

We can do the same with our earnings. What are our most enjoyable ways to make money? It makes sense to focus our efforts on these as we'll have more energy and enthusiasm to do the work.

20/10 – Are you a perfectionist?

Several years ago, someone told me she hadn't realised I was a perfectionist. I felt that, in not being more easily recognised as one, I was a *failure* as perfectionist. And then I laughed at myself.

This is another common subpersonality **(10/1)** which is often associated with shame and failure. After all, perfection for humans doesn't exist. We can befriend our perfectionism, noticing what triggers it. What that part of us needs. How it's actually trying to help us.

And then we can reframe our efforts so we make it at least a possibility (more likely with planning) that we'll reach our goals.

21/10 – There's more to you than whatever you're dealing with

When something's taking up a lot of headspace - from a health condition to an issue with a neighbour, financial woes to missing an ex, grief to trauma and anxiety - it's easy to get caught up in the drama of it all.

Psychosynthesis, a transpersonal psychology, recognises that there's a part of us that's already whole. Whatever we're struggling with, no matter how all-encompassing it may feel, there is so much more to us that that.

Remembering this can help us access more of our resources **(15/10)** as well as making it easier to tune into that wise, whole part of ourselves **(25/2)**.

187

22/10 – Retraining our autonomic nervous system (ANS)

While we do certain things (like breathe) automatically, changing our breath **(9/1)** for just a few minutes can change our physiology. Calming breaths mean the calmer, more relaxed signals going up to our brains via the vagus nerve **(29/2)** and then coming back down to the whole system.

The initial yoga therapy training I did was based around retraining the ANS through yoga and pranayama. Lifting (energising) then lowering (calming) the ANS through breaths like Ujjayi **(6/4)** followed by Kapalabhati **(23/2)** and dynamic movement like Sun Salutations followed by Savasana **(26/10)** help us get used to that lifting and lowering on the yoga mat.

With practice, this retrains the ANS. Emotional stresses that would have been very lifting in the past, become far more manageable as we have greater heart rate variability. This boosts our emotional and physiological resilience as well as our heart health.

23/10 – Being open to guidance

As part of my morning meditations, I ask my Miraculous Self **(27/3)** to guide my every interaction, action, even email. Some days, I'm better at paying attention to the guidance I receive than others.

Some people pray, others meditate, others tune into that wise part of themselves while out running, swimming, fishing or whatever works for them.

If you believe in God, Goddess, the Universe, saints and angels or simply a part of you that's beyond the everyday and knows the best step in any situation, don't be shy about asking.

24/10 – Listening to our wisest selves

As above (23/10), some days this is easier than others. While not especially practical for every day, when the pool is fairly quiet*, I do what I call Angel Stroke. Floating slowly on my back, gliding my arms through the water as if making a snow angel, I mentally think of an old prayer, 'Mother Goddess, Father God, Angels, Guides and Helpers, lead me today and every day to my highest good. I am open to miracles.'

Sometimes, 'answers' pop into my head. Other times, I feel nothing but impatience at how slow the stroke is. This is a sure sign, with hindsight, that I would benefit from slowing down and being more receptive and open.

What conditions most help you?

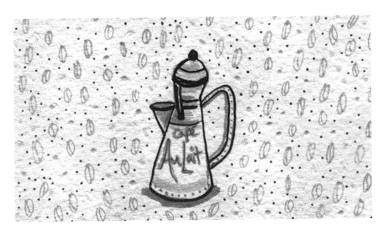

25/10 – Clocks falling back

As we gain an extra hour, as well as pondering how best to luxuriate in it, go further.

Imagine a whole extra day. Unscheduled. No demands. Imagine you've already caught up on all your sleep debt.

What would you do with a free day?

Imagine it in detail. What time, who with and where would you like to wake up? What about breakfast, your free morning, lunch, afternoon, evening and dinner? The night? Be as specific as possible.

---

* or, even better, in the sea.

Are there any themes? What elements might you take from your imaginary free day to infuse everyday with more freedom?

26/10 – Savasana

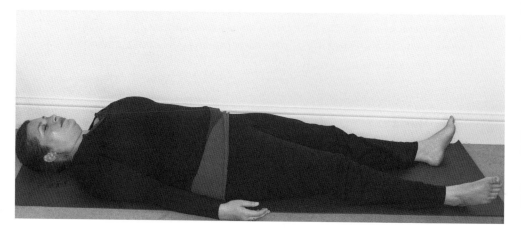

If you struggle in Savasana, maybe knowing the physiological benefits will encourage you to persevere. Its capacity to retrain the ANS **(22/10)** so we're better able to calm ourselves down off the yoga mat as well as during our practice can motivate us. And if, like many, you already enjoy it, I hope you'll appreciate it even more knowing just how good it is for us.

We spend a lot of time rushing about, pushing ourselves to accomplish more and more. Our nervous systems rarely need any help in being lifted; this 24/7 society does that for us. An email (or even a *thought* about an email – or anything else) can trigger the same stress response **(3/4)** that our ancient ancestors reserved for genuine threats to their lives.

✓ To practice (don't be fooled – it may look simple but it *is* a practice – some days will feel easier than others), lie on your mat with your head, neck and spine nicely aligned. Allow the feet and legs to roll out and release the arms away from the body with the palms facing up.

- ✓ If there's any discomfort, a bolster, cushion or rolled up blankets under your knees can ease that.
- ✓ Tune into your own body's wisdom to see if there's anything else you need in this moment. Maybe a blanket, socks, whatever might make you more comfortable as you allow the benefits of your yoga practice (or run, or any other type of exertion) to sink in.

While it may be easy for you to simply let go and relax, using the breath as an anchor **(7/1)** can minimise rumination, stressful thoughts and flashbacks. You'll probably notice that it's much easier to practice after a more dynamic session than simply going from being quite inactive to Savasana. Movement helps to burn off lots of the stress hormones, allowing the system to release that anxiety and stress. Notice the heart rate, breath, the feel of the ground supporting you and so on.

If you're still feeling a bit antsy, you might want to co-ordinate the tightening and releasing of the thighs **(15/8)** with each breath (inhale tighten, exhale release). As well as offering a focus for your mind, this honours the body's natural fight/flight impulse (relaxation can trigger that when it hasn't felt safe to relax). Using the larger muscles in the thighs can burn off more of those stress hormones.

You might also want to use the time to release unhelpful habits, behaviours, beliefs, aches, pains, tensions, stresses and worries into the earth. It can all be recycled for the benefit of the planet.

You may consciously think, 'Yup, defo ready to release _____!' or it may be a more general, trusting, letting go of whatever's ready to be let go of without even consciously remembering it.

As with everything, you know yourself best and what's best for you during any given practice.

27/10 – Prudence

Not just a character in *Charmed*, this Universal Strength **(31/5)** allows us to restrain ourselves, apply Wisdom **(11/9)** and make good decisions. It can help us on a path of moderation but, to our hedonistic twenty-first century eyes can often seem quite old fashioned.

Overplayed we might become over cautious and penny pinching. Underplayed, we can throw caution to the wind and end up in debt - or overweight or drunk or whatever our particular issue is.

How might you be more prudent today?

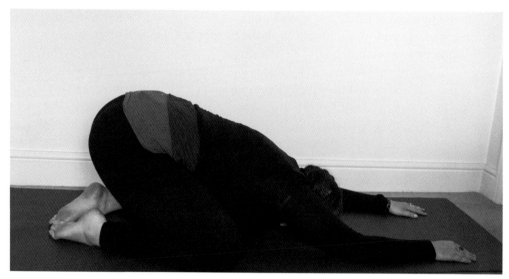

28/10 – Child pose

Child is said to be especially good when menstruating. Mukunda Stiles, in *Structural Yoga Therapy* (Goodwill, 2002) writes that it can help eliminate extra fluid and energy. Along with stress relief, benefits include stretching the spine, hips, thighs and ankles. It should be avoided if you are pregnant, have diarrhoea or if knee issues make it uncomfortable.

Child can also encourage self-care. Even with a yoga instructor reminding us to feel free to relax into Child anytime we choose, we're still likely to pause as we watch what everyone else is doing. Yet learning to choose what's right for us in any given moment is liberating and empowering.

Notice Child variations. Sometimes, the outstretched arms feel best. Other times, you may want to rest with the hands as a pillow for your forehead (see below) or even wrapped around your torso, first resting on one temple and then gently turning so both sides of the neck feel balanced.

If you want to play with Child pose, while it's traditionally taught with the knees together, many adults simply aren't shaped that way. You may want to kneel with your knees wide apart and big toes together. This will allow you to relax more deeply into Child than attempting to keep the buttocks on the heels as your forehead reaches for the mat (of course, if your body does work that way and you find this relaxing, go for it!).

We can also use Child pose to consciously release any headaches and heart aches into the earth, knowing they can be recycled for the benefit of the planet.

29/10 – Does life keep spooking you? Try Bhu mudra

I learned this mudra **(3/5)** from Nancy Jean Mirales (www.yourbeautiful chakras.com). It's brilliant for grounding yourself when you're sitting down.

Make the peace sign with both hands and bring the thumb and other fingers together. Connect the peace sign fingers to the ground next to you

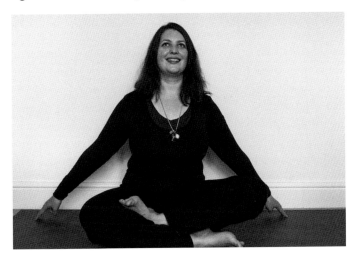

so your arms, long and straight, create the slopes of a mountain and your crown is the peak.

Mentally (or aloud if you want to) affirm 'My roots ground deep into the heart of the living earth.' Allow yourself to feel the support of the earth.

30/10 – Befriending our inner monsters

Hallowe'en is a brilliant opportunity to embrace our inner monsters. Whether you're choosing a fancy dress costume or just imagining one, notice what you're most drawn to.

What are your monster's (or any costume you can think of) superpowers?

What is its shadow side?

What does your choice tell you about yourself and what you want more or less of year-round?

31/10 – Samhain/Hallowe'en

Parties aside, this is a great time of year to reflect on people and animals who've passed on. It's believed to be the time of year where the veil between living and dead is thinnest. We don't need to be morbid to pause to honour our ancestors and loved ones. Think about the impact they've had on you and celebrate their lives.

It's also a great time of year to remind ourselves that no matter how depressing things can seem, it will get brighter. We can have fun again. We can release what we're ready to let go of and move on with wisdom, honouring those who came before us by living as well as possible ourselves. We can also ponder the kind of legacy we want to leave for those who'll come after us. Do we want to leave them to clear up our mess or can we make the world a bit better before we leave it?

November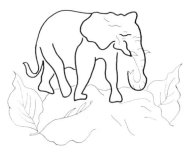

This month's tips include some holistic goal setting support, ways to bring more joy, kindness and compassion into our lives and exploring the times criticisms simply don't land.

1/11 – The veil between our worlds

While Samhain **(31/10)** is very much about honouring our natural grief and loss, the world we live in sometimes pathologises such natural processes. People used to wear black for a year. Things stopped. For some, this was repressive but now, for many, we've gone too far in the opposite direction. Some feel there's something wrong with them when of *course* it can take longer than a few weeks, months or years.

Whatever you're feeling is perfectly natural. A therapist can help you process the grief and loss but, most importantly, *you* can honour however you feel. There may be days when you feel guilty about laughing, smiling or looking ahead. Other time, maybe you can't imagine any of that.

Be extra kind to yourself, whatever you're feeling.

2/11 – What is the elephant in the room?

That issue that you're determined to ignore no matter how much energy it takes to do so?

What springs to mind? What colour is the elephant? How big is it? Is it friendly or fierce? What does it represent? A relationship? An issue at work? Something family related? A trauma you've survived? An addiction?

Our elephants have become elephants because we're scared. From a resourceful state of mind **(15/10)**, what springs to mind as a potential baby step you could take towards dealing with your elephant?

How might you put supports in place to help you handle it as easily as possible?

3/11 – Changing our perception

This NLP tool, based on Gestallt chair work, is known as Perceptual Positions.

- ✓ Taking three chairs, name one 'You', another '[Whoever your issue is with]' and the third, 'the Observer' or 'your Higher/Miraculous Self' **(27/3)**.
- ✓ Sitting in the You chair, you can whinge about the situation to our heart's content. Afterwards, you can stand and Taylor Swift (Shake it Off) before sitting in the Whoever chair and noticing what emerges from this vantage point.
- ✓ You might go back and forth from You to Whoever several times as you build on the insights this can offer.
- ✓ When ready to take the Observer chair, notice what comes up here. Maybe you want to go back to You or Whoever or maybe you're done.

Repeat as needed, remembering to step into a neutral spot to shake off each position before taking the next.

4/11 – Yoga and a flexible mind

Yoga poses such as Triangle **(1/2)** - or anything that has us view the world from an unusual angle - can help us see our issues in a new light.

We experience our practices differently depending on the room or outdoor space we see each time. We can experiment.

With practice, it's natural to improve our flexibility of mind as well as of body, and, of course, strength and stamina.

5/11 – Anchoring good feelings

Anchors **(8/5)**, in NLP, are ways to physically reconnect with an emotion or state (confidence, joy, peace, resourcefulness, whatever) with ease. We can remember a time we felt what we want to recreate and make it as vivid as possible. By sensing into it, we embody it again and once we're done, we anchor it by, for example, touching thumb and middle finger together or holding the left earlobe.

Similar to mudras **(3/5)**, anchors can be very discreet. This makes them easy to replicate at work, on a plane or during that family dinner.

The more we do it, the stronger the associations grow and the more deeply we can sense into those good feelings.

6/11 – Making space for a practice that suits you

When I used to read about people's meditative practices, I'd inwardly roll my eyes. Yet I now depend on my own so much that even on my earliest mornings (rare, thankfully), I'll set my alarm earlier in order to fit it in with a little yoga.

Each summer, I hop on a train to the coast once a week. I work many evenings and Saturdays so carving out a morning each week is one of my biggest acts of self-care and totally worth it. Year-round, if I don't make it to the pool at least twice a week, I start feeling like an amoeba.

What spiritual, physical and emotional practices help you meet the demands of your everyday life?

How can you prioritise them more?

7/11 – Oxytocin and reaching out

This 'care hormone' is boosted in breastfeeding mothers. For the rest of us, we can enhance it through connecting with others, skin to skin contact and even wishing others well. Unfortunately, our oxytocin levels drop when we feel disconnected from others. This heightens our feelings of isolation, potentially creating a vicious circle where we withdraw further.

Learning this on my initial yoga therapy training felt pretty transformative and, along with Elena's advice **(12/10)** has been a healing practice.

When you think of the upcoming holidays, who do you most look forward to engaging with and reaching out to or welcoming into your home?

8/11 – Who do you most like spending time with?

As above, these connections are good for our health. Obviously, there'll always be people who we might doubt have any positive impact on our oxytocin levels **(7/11)**.

By being aware of who we most enjoy spending time with, we're better able to make them a bigger part of our lives. This will help us be better company with the people we might not choose to spend time with.

Making time for a good level - we're all different - of alone time can help, too.

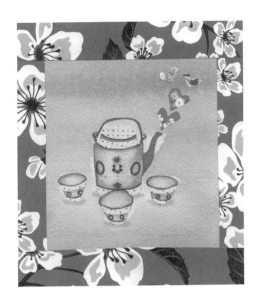

9/11 – What do you most like doing?

When we have a better understanding of the tasks that energise us, we can schedule more of them in. Looking at our diaries for the coming day or week (or mentally scanning our plans), we immediately get a sense of what we're looking forward to or dreading.

We can notice certain patterns. With work (as far as possible) and our own time (again, recognising some limitations), how might we make more time to do the things we most love?

10/11 – What do we least like doing?

What stands out as your biggest 'Urgh' as you imagine your day or week ahead?

Many people think we need to be positive all the time. Yet recognising what *doesn't* work for us is valuable information. We can use our pain, frustration and irritation to make changes that create more congruent harmony. When thinking of our biggest 'Urghs', one may spring to mind or an instant list might emerge.

Either way, whether working with one or several, we can notice ways to minimise them as much as possible.

11/11 – What can you cancel?

Obviously, it's not *always* possible to clear the joyless from our lives but, often, it is. When you think of the coming twenty-four hours, can anything be delegated or simply cancelled?

I'm not suggesting we stop doing the things people depend on us for. What about the little things that don't make a difference yet drain our energy?

What springs to mind?

12/11 – What sparks the most joy amongst your day to day tasks and habits?

What do you appreciate most about your everyday life?

What makes your heart sing?

How can you do more of these things?

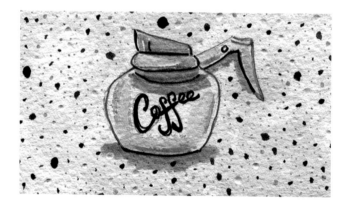

13/11 – Happy World Kindness Day!

While we normally think of kindness in relation to others, the better care we take of ourselves, the more kindness and patience we have for others.

What would extra kindness look like for yourself today?

How about for a loved one?

How about for a stranger?

Colleague?

Someone you feel challenged by?

Even sending loving kindness **(15/2)** when we feel helpless can help boost the world's kindness levels. And it has a ripple effect.

14/11 – Kindness

Kindness is another Universal Strength **(31/5)**. Ellen DeGeneres is known for her catchphrase, 'Be kind to one another' and Piero Ferrucci's gorgeous *The Power of Kindness* (Penguin, 2006) is a meditation on its benefits. As Maya Angelou famously said, we might forget what people did but we never forget how they made us feel.

While kindness costs nothing, I notice that I'm far more likely to be kind when my self-care is good. When I'm running on empty, I'm less likely to hold that door open for a stranger or put myself out for others' benefit. Overplayed, kindness can be cloying. It's like the old joke about the Girl Scout helping the elderly lady across the road before checking she *wanted* to cross. It can also feed into our Martyr subpersonality **(10/1)** tendencies.

Underplayed, we think only of ourselves and life gets much harsher and colder, not just for those we're less kind (or even unkind) to but for ourselves.

How might you be kinder – to yourself *and* others – today?

15/11 – Wheel

Just as forward folds are typically calming*, backbends help energise us and can improve our mood.

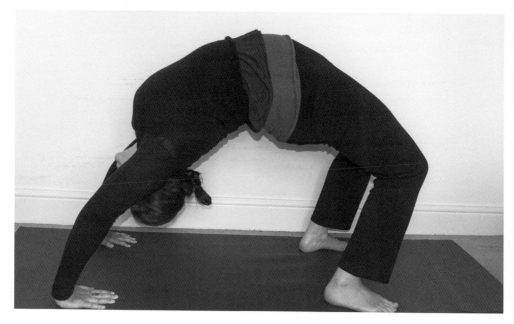

Do this towards the end of your practice when you're warmed up (injuring yourself is unlikely to improve your mood). Sun Salutations warm the whole body while Chair, Equestrian and Pigeon target the larger muscles in the legs.

Starting with Bridge pose **(11/3)**, a great backbend on its own, once your spine feels warmed up and if you feel like continuing into Wheel, lie back down onto your back and bring the hands over your shoulders and into position for Wheel.

You may want to stay there. Check in with yourself at every step and if you're not familiar with yoga or have any injuries or hesitations, don't do this without support or supervision. If you want to continue, lift the hips and come onto the crown of your head, pausing. If it feels good for your body, come up into the full pose.

---

*not for everyone – the more you practice, the better you'll get to know your *own* body and what works best for *you*.

202

Notice what's happening with your breath, aiming to continue breathing fully and deeply for as long as feels comfortable. It may be one complete breath, maybe five. You know yourself best.

When you come back down, notice what's happening with your mouth. Are you smiling? Notice however it is you're feeling.

It may be that coming *out* of the pose is what lifts your mood but it's a great one to play with if Wheel appeals. It can also help us retrain our nervous systems over time, increasing our allostatic load which, in turn, helps us better manage bigger stresses *off* the yoga mat.

You can get many of the benefits by mimicking the pose over a Swiss ball. This way, you're opening the body in the same way but don't have to support all of your weight with your arms and legs.

16/11 – Tree

Brilliant for grounding and balance, Tree is a wonderful barometer for our concentration. Some days, it may feel effortless. Other times, our thoughts get in the way, we lose focus and our balance.

The vestibular system is influenced by our emotions. The kinder we can be to ourselves if we fall out of Tree, the easier it is to rebalance and bring ourselves back up. If you lose your balance, pause to reground before coming back up again.

As well as aiding physical balance and centring the mind, Tree is great for boosting concentration. Start with a minute on each side (or a few seconds – start where you are. It'll come with practice) and aim to build up to holding it for five minutes on each side.

From Mountain pose, focus your eyes on something still. Feel the soles of the feet supported by the mat and ground below you. Imagine growing roots from the foot you're going to start with, going deep into the earth and supporting you.

Allow your weight to go more into this first foot and when you feel ready, keeping your hips square and even, lift the other foot to the ankle, calf or thigh (not on the knee as you don't want to put pressure on the joint).

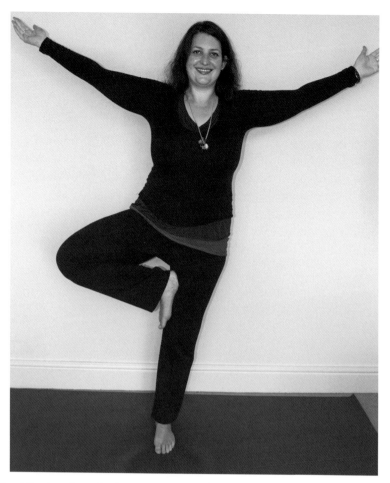

Rest the hands at the heart centre or above the head. Again, notice which variation helps you feel most balanced.

Even if you feel like you're low, you'll really notice results if you keep practicing. Build up from a place of strength, grounding and balance.

Use all available resources, too. As well as keeping your eyes focused on something still, use a wall or chair or similar for support if needed.

I love the beams at the Feel Better Every Day Consultancy. It's a Grade II listed building so they're slightly wonky but it's great to have that tree energy in the space. If you have high blood pressure, avoid the arms outstretched like branches above your head variation.

Tree offers a great way to wake up the body, imagining the sun's healing rays pouring into your leaves and branches. If you have insomnia, avoid Tree in the late afternoon or evening.

17/11 – The logical levels

Also known as neurological levels, this is one of my favourite NLP tools. Created by Robert Dilts, it helps us embody various levels of change. We can examine our goals **(13/10)** from several different angles and sense into each level.

The following days **(18/11 -23/11)** go into more detail about each one. To start, consider a goal (aka well-formed outcome **(7/10)**).

Ideally, we physically step into each one (we can use a piece of paper with the level jotted down and move up and down the levels). It can be illuminating and really shifts energy around our goals.

18/11 – Environment

Stepping onto the first level, when you think of working towards your goal **(17/11)**, and you consider your environment, does it feel supportive? Is it sabotaging you? For example, if you want to make healthier food choices, is your kitchen filled with cakes and other obstacles to healthy eating?

Would filling it with fresh fruits and veg (leaving room for cakes as treats, perhaps) help?

Maybe your goal is to bring more life into your work/life balance. Has your home office taken over your living room?

Whatever your goal, notice what springs to mind when you consider the environment you're mostly in when working towards it. What tweaks might better support you?

Environment can include our clothing, shoes, car and more.

19/11 – Behaviour

Once we've looked at our Environment **(18/11)**, we step forward to Behaviour. From this spot, what springs to mind as we consider our current behaviour affecting this goal **(17/11)**?

What are we doing that brings us closer?

What might be sabotaging ourselves? Some work with our Saboteur **(19/1)** may be useful.

What essential behaviours are we skipping?

How can we better support ourselves in doing more of what will work?

20/11 – Skills and capabilities

Sometimes, our Environment **(18/11)** and Behaviour **(19/11)** is stuck because we simply don't know *how* to do better. As Maya Angelou famously said, 'Once you knew better, you did better'.

Is there a way to get more training to get you through this patch?

Maybe it's just a matter of asking someone and tapping into your resourcefulness **(15/10)**. What springs to mind as you contemplate your goal from the Skills and Capabilities spot?

21/11 – Beliefs and values

Sometimes, our Beliefs and Values are at odds with our goals. Even if we're doing all the right things (and know how to) in the right places, if we're fundamentally at odds with ourselves, we'll keep sabotaging ourselves.

As you step from Skills and Capabilities **(20/11)** to Beliefs and Values, what springs to mind?

Which values support you in your pursuit of your goal **(17/11)** and which get in your way?

What do you realise about yourself and your goal as you ponder this?

22/11 – Identity

For my first several years as a coach, there was a discrepancy between my coaching work and my idea of how a 'proper coach' would be. While I adore what I do, I'm not a corporate soul. And my style, while challenging when needed, is also gentle.

Adding other therapies helped and I'm quick (and happy) to refer people on if they call and sound like they need someone more dynamic. My normal work environment (a beamed room in a Grade II listed property with nods to Ganesh, Mary, Buddha, Lakshmi and the brain) is perfect for my integrative practice.

Now, when I go into organisations, because my focus is very much on embodied self-care, there's no incongruence.

What springs to mind for you as you step from Beliefs and Values **(21/11)** to Identity?

23/11 – Spirituality/purpose

This is the game changer. Where we step beyond our own little world into something bigger. If we believe in God/Goddess, the Universe or any kind of spirituality, this can enhance our sense of purpose **(7/12)**.

If we don't, simply tuning into that highest, wisest, most miraculous part of ourselves **(27/3)** can help us tune into a sense of motivation **(9/3)** we never knew existed.

What springs to mind as you step from Identity **(22/11)** and ponder your goal from this space of Purpose?

What happens as you think about some of the obstacles that have sprung to mind as you've tuned into each level?

24/11 – Going back through each level

When you feel ready, turn around and look back. From this space of embodied Purpose, walk back through each level.

How do you feel about your Identity **(22/11)** now you can integrate that higher, more spiritual energy?

How about your Beliefs and Values **(21/11)** now you have the added insights regarding your Identity and Purpose **(23/11)**?

And as you step back to Skills and Capabilities **(20/11)**, what else can you bring to your pondering here?

How about your Behaviour **(19/11)**? Does this feel easier to change now you have more insight?

And your Environment **(18/11)**? What changes are you ready to make to better support yourself as you work towards this goal?

Making notes can help us ground this. Scheduling any concrete actions in can help us build on our insights.

25/11 – The pons and posture

How are you sitting right now? I'm drafting this hunched over my tablet, sending my brain even stronger signals than usual (when hunched over my laptop) that I feel like prey. Even though, consciously, I feel fine, my brain is sending signals, via the pons, to the rest of my system, based on this posture it interprets as fearful.

If I didn't counter unhealthy work postures with lots of expansive **(26/11)** swimming, yoga and mini trampoline 'dancing', it would have a greater impact on my confidence and assertiveness. Amy Cuddy calls it the iHunch and the smaller our devices, the more fearful our posture becomes and the less assertively we act.

How do you feel when you stand or sit up straighter? What happens to your breath **(7/1)**? How about your mood?

26/11 – Power poses

I've mentioned Amy Cuddy's *Presence: Bringing your Boldest Self to Your Biggest Challenges* (Little, Brown and Company, 2015) many times **(13/2, 18/2, 20/2, 22/6, 19/7, 23/7, 12/10** and **25/11). Her** work is revolutionary *and* incredibly easy to put into practice to bring enormous benefits. If you haven't seen her TED Talk on how changing our posture can change our lives, you can view it here: https://www.ted.com/talks/amy_cuddy_your_body_language_shapes_who_you_are?language=en

In a nutshell, Cuddy was motivated by her own recovery from a traumatic brain injury. She also wanted to help her Harvard Business School students who knew their stuff but weren't presenting well. She and her colleagues, Dana Carney and Andy Yap, measured cortisol and testosterone levels before and after two minutes' power posing (think Wonder Woman, Superman a starfish, Warrior II or any expansive posture). Afterwards, cortisol levels (stress) dropped and testosterone (confidence) increased. This gave participants a greater sense of being in their own power (sacral **(10/7)**).

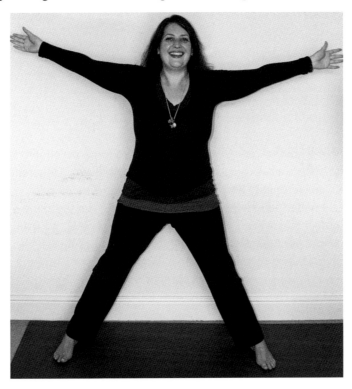

Beyond their own perceptions, a panel of fake job interviewers rated the power pose group as more competent saying they'd choose those participants.

The benefit can last for hours and I've also heard of people power posing in carparks and at work.

27/11 - The heart's electromagnetic field

HeartMath Institute research shows that our heart's electromagnetic field expands when we meditate on peace, love and kindness. Metta is wonderful **(15/2)** but anytime we send someone good wishes, we are strengthening our own hearts as well as helping the wider world. Kok et al. (2013, *Psychological Science*) found it helps us feel more connected to others.

Taking care of ourselves, by grounding, centring **(13/3)** and coherent breathing are some of the best things we can do for all concerned.

28/11 - Pendulum effect on others

Researchers from the HeartMath Institute encourage psychophysiological coherence with their biofeedback tools like emWave. Coherence is not relaxation, as we're still alert and our functioning is increased.

Just as smaller pendulums will fall in line with the largest, by stepping into our power and staying centred and grounded **(13/3)**, we can influence those around us to tap into their own coherence and centred presence.

We can do this in meetings, in the car, on a plane, in a lift or at a dinner. Anytime we notice group energy getting a bit frazzled, by pausing to look after our own energy, we can really shift things for the better.

29/11 – Dehydroepiandrosterone (DHEA)

Produced in the adrenal glands, DHEA (dehydroepiandrosterone) is a performance enhancer. Banned in athletics when taken orally, we can create it naturally. DHEA is created using the same building blocks as cortisol. This means that when we're feeling great and producing DHEA, we're unable to create cortisol.

Positive emotions (like joy **(12/11)**, hope **(11/6)**, love **(3/12)**, pride **(3/7)**, awe **(5/12)**) not only feel good as we experience them but last for hours physiologically by boosting DHEA.

Happy Place meditations **(17/12)** can be a way to cultivate these good feelings no matter what's actually going on. This then helps us tune into our resources **(15/10)** and tweak things to improve our situation.

30/11 – Purple elephant syndrome

It's so easy to ignore all the positive feedback we get from the world (sensory acuity **(8/10)**) and tune into that one negative comment. Yet certain criticisms, no matter how strong our self-loathing inner critic **(3/10)**, simply don't resonate.

For most of us, being called a purple elephant is one of these things. We *know* we're not purple. And even when we've been over eating, we mostly know we're not elephants.

Which kind of criticisms knock you off balance?

Which wash over you because there's no part of you that gives it power?

Observing our inner critic in this way may feel a little scary but can be very illuminating.

December

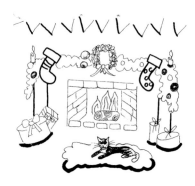

This month's tips include self-indulgently good, natural ways to create a performance enhancing drug, energetic self-defence, a Hawaiian reconciliation and forgiveness meditation and some ways to end the year well.

1/12 – World AIDS Day

Apart from the obvious safe sex reminders, this awareness day reminds us of the power of destigmatising. While much remains to be done, we've come a long way in just a few decades.

www.worldaidsday.org gives more information about ways we can spread hope rather than ignorance. One day, this disease will be a thing of the past.

2/12 – Ways to boost DHEA

We can help our bodies produce more DHEA **(29/11)** by consciously taking time to cultivate the feelings that have been proven to boost it. When do you naturally feel more joy **(12/11)**, hope **(11/6)**, love **(3/12)**, pride **(3/7)**, awe **(5/12)** and so on?

Even when we don't have time to physically do something, we can meditate on it to give our bodies a taste of how it feels. This can help us look forward to planned DHEA boosting activities as well as getting a taste in advance.

How might you make more time to do these things?

3/12 – Love

One of the main archetypes in psychosynthesis (along with the Will **(15/6)**), Love is also a Universal Strength **(31/5)**. Love helps us connect to our loved ones, ourselves, strangers, colleagues and even people on the other side of the world. Love helps us feel safe and expansive.

Overplayed, we might find ourselves in love with the *idea* of Love, pursuing less healthy relationships by talking ourselves into them. We might feel taken advantage of.

Underplayed, we can feel isolated and disconnected.

Feeling Love, be it for a child, animal, lover, family member, stranger, place or anything at all, boosts our DHEA levels **(2/12)**. We're reducing stress and helping our immune function as well as performance.

How might you be more loving today?

4/12 – Energetic self defence

There are lots of things we can do to protect our energy fields and spaces. Visualising ourselves surrounded by a protective white cloak or bubble, using symbols and crystals **(22/8)** are just a few. One of my favourite tools is Giser's space clearing **(2/1)**. While we're releasing energies that aren't authentically ours, we're also supporting our Miraculous Self and clearing the path ahead.

I like Giser's encouragement to bring other energies in. They may be grounding and protective, they may be glittery and expansive. Whatever feels best. This can feel gentler and more optimistic than some of the protective meditations as we're automatically thinking of things we need to protect ourselves from.

Focusing on what we want tends to be more powerful than worrying about what we don't want.

5/12 – Awe and Appreciation

Another DHEA **(2/12)** boosting emotion, as identified by the HeartMath Institute, Awe allows us to appreciate beauty and excellence (another Universal Strength **(31/5)**). Awe can connect us with the miraculous in life, from watching Olympians and Paralympians to losing ourselves in piece of art, Awe inspires us to do better.

Overplayed, we might figure there's no *way* we can come anywhere near such magnificence in our own endeavours. Why even bother?

Underplayed, we can become cynical. Instead of appreciating the beauty of nature, we might litter and pollute.

How might you bring more Awe into your day?

6/12 – More on DHEA

DHEA **(2/12)** is often known as a youth or vitality hormone. We produce more when we're younger and continue to produce it when we're energised by positive emotions.

The emWave from the HeartMath Institute (www.heartmath.org) helps us see the impact of shifting our thoughts from stressful ones to accessing positive emotions and memories.

With practice, we can bring more coherence to our brains and hearts, supporting the whole system and helping us feel better.

7/12 – Spirituality (purpose) universal strength

Whether we identify as being spiritual, religious or simply feel a sense of purpose, this universal strength **(31/5)** can help give meaning to our lives. Especially when things feel challenging.

Overplayed, it may mean trying to rush through perfectly natural, human feelings in an effort to embody 'love and light'. We might project our own anger and rage onto others. We might shame ourselves for taking time to recover before getting to the post-traumatic growth bit.

In balance, we can recognise whatever human experience our spirit is having (no matter how painful). We can also look out for whatever's trying to emerge, what we can learn and how we can grow from it.

How might you make space for your spirit to guide you today?

8/12 – Common senses

In almost any guided meditation (including yoga nidra **(9/3)**), there'll be elements of using our senses to go deeper. I learned about VAKOG (the five main senses we interpret the world through) during my NLP training.

V - visual (seeing)
A - auditory (hearing)
K - kinaesthetic (feeling, both physiologically and emotionally)
O - olfactory (smelling) and
G - gustatory (tasting).

We all have preferences so, for example, some of us learn better through experiencing (kinaesthetic), listening or reading. I'm sure Joan Wilmot's delicious cakes (gustatory and olfactory) helped us learn more on our clinical supervision training.

We can consciously use all our senses any time. When we tune into our Happy Place **(17/12)** and DHEA boosting emotions **(2/12)**, we can allow ourselves to deepen the experience by noticing what we see, hear, feel, smell and taste.

Christiane Sanderson **(30/6)** recommends creating a physical Mood Box, incorporating something from each sense so we can instantly grab a smell (herbal tea bag, essential oil, perfume or whatever appeals to you), taste (something that won't go off), picture, music or sound and maybe nice fabric or something else pleasantly tactile to feel.

9/12 – Self-care boost

If you could do one little thing to support yourself a little better, what might it be?

What kind of lifestyle would feel better (just imagining for now, as if money were no object)?

What kind of holiday might feel like just what the doctor ordered?

How about an ideal weekend to give you a new lease of life?

Just one day, even an afternoon or hour spent in a way to soothe your soul?

What would help you take better care of yourself with whatever time you *can* carve out for yourself?

10/12 – Happy International Mountain Day!

Which mountain, real or metaphorical is your Everest? What feels like a sometimes impossible dream but keeps bubbling up? Maybe performing stand-up comedy? Singing in public? Writing a book? Going to university or retraining in a different field? Trekking Machu Pichu? Actually climbing a mountain? Building a house? What springs to mind for you?

11/12 – What might be a first step up this mountain?

Now you're fired up about the spectacular views awaiting you at the top of your metaphorical or actual mountain, what is a baby step you feel excited about taking?

As the old saying goes, we don't need to be able to see the whole staircase, just our next step.

12/12 – Imposter syndrome

The term Imposter Phenomenon was coined by Pauline Clance and Suzanne Imes in their seminal 1978 paper. It describes the way we can feel fraudulent and inadequate no matter how well we are doing. Decades later, it's still relevant. I interviewed Dr Valerie Young a few years ago after she published her book, *The Secret Thoughts of Successful Women – Why Capable People Suffer from the Imposter Syndrome and How to Thrive in Spite of It* (Crown, 2011).

It affects most men, too. We're in good company: Maya Angelou, Mike Myers, Kate Winslet and Meryl Streep are just a few who've struggled with it. I especially appreciated Young's description of herself as a 'recovering imposter'.

Knowing the phenomenon exists doesn't make us immune. Recognising that certain situations will trigger such feelings mean we can build in more support for ourselves when we're likely to feel more wobbly. This is especially important during times when we're most likely to feel triggered, such as being part of a minority group, living abroad, studying and starting a new job. Young says it takes at least six months in a new role for most people even though we often expect ourselves to hit the ground running.

Professors and 'experts' can support others by voicing our own histories with Imposter Syndrome. As Valerie told me, it affects just about anyone who's been 'raised by humans'.

13/12 – Resolution Magic stomping

I learned this from Olivia Roberts, author of *Chronic Pain and Debilitating Conditions Resolution* (Findhorn Press, 2012) at an energy therapy conference a few years ago. It sounds silly but is an incredibly effective way of shifting energy, releasing anger and honouring whatever is upsetting us. In a nutshell, when we can't be bothered to tap **(8/8)** and have the space and privacy to do this, we can stamp our feet, pump our arms and shout 'Go away!'

The issue could be an unresolved argument, something on the news, recurring stressful thoughts, a one off stressful thought or physical ailment. Olivia developed this as a way to manage migraines and IBS. We're essentially changing the way we feel by using our bodies **(29/2)**. Sometimes, a few stamps and shouts has us laughing and fine. Others, we may wind ourselves up and realise the situation is more upsetting than we've realised.

By honouring the fight flight impulse **(3/4)** as well as our voices, we empower ourselves to make practical changes to the situation, too.

14/12 – More on oxytocin and ways to boost it

Known as the 'care hormone', oxytocin **(7/11)** is released when we fall in love, through breast feeding and when we connect. According to Dr Paul Zak, author of *The Moral Molecule* (Corgi, 2013), we also release it through hugs and handshakes when they're genuinely warm with eye contact. And apparently, all the tears I've shed over films and books have been boosting my oxytocin levels, too! Any kind of connection (even with fictional characters) can help.

So does singing **(2/3)** with other people, like at karaoke or in a choir or band. Similarly, dancing, rollercoaster/bungee and seeing a horror film with someone else. In spite of social media's bad rap, Zak found that levels of oxytocin rise after people checked Facebook and twitter, although, obviously, it doesn't replace real contact.

Treating loved ones (from a full cup, not if we're running on empty) and even telling them we love them can also boost oxytocin, helping us connect and feel connected.

15/12 – Serotonin

This neurotransmitter boosts our wellbeing and happiness. It helps us grow, aids memory and learning, regulates mood, appetite, sleep and impacts willpower **(12/4)** and delaying gratification. This is why, sometimes, we can't do the simplest seeming things when we've exerted ourselves to complete a big project).

'It is estimated that 90 per cent of the body's serotonin is actually made in the digestive tract,' says Natalie Lamb, nutritionist at www.bio-kult.com. 'Its production by cells in the intestinal lining is highly influenced by certain bacteria there. Recent studies have shown that low serotonin production can be reversed when the gut flora is rebalanced. Consuming fermented foods and/or live bacterial probiotic supplements has been shown to help rebalance gut bacteria.'

According to *Psychology Today* blogger, Dr Alex Korb, we can also boost serotonin levels with sunlight. Vitamin D helps boost our mood because it promotes serotonin production. Massage and other human contact also help.

Thinking of positive memories increases serotonin production in the anterior cingulate cortex. Focusing on sad memories decreases serotonin production in same part of brain. Choosing our mental focus, literally choosing happy thoughts, not only boosts serotonin but gives our brains and bodies a break from the effects of those sadder thoughts.

Exercise can boost serotonin but only when we genuinely *want* to do it. Yoga helps as do aerobic exercises such as cycling and running. Korb suggests that the body can somehow differentiate between running for our lives, when being hunted, and running for fun.

Enjoying our exercise makes it even better for us.

16/12 – Dopamine

This feel good hormone is a neurotransmitter that gets released by the anticipation of reward. When we have lots of dopamine, as well as feeling good, we're motivated. Certain drugs become addictive because they trigger dopamine release. The faster the release, the more addictive the substance. We can boost dopamine by doing things like yoga nidra **(9/3)** as well as putting rewards (of various sizes depending on what they're for) in place and making sure we follow through and enjoy the fruits of our labours.

Dopamine can also be boosted by a message from someone we hope to hear from and can make our devices and social media quite addictive **(18/9)**.

17/12 – Happy place

Sometimes known as a 'safe place' meditation, this can then make it feel like other places are *un*safe so use the term that feels best for you. I learned this on my initial yoga therapy training.

We can either remember or imagine a time when we felt completely at ease, embodied, happy and well. It may have been years ago or earlier today. You may have lots of memories or it may be something you're imagining *could* feel happy and at ease.

Whatever springs to mind, allow yourself to relax into the memory or imagining. How does it feel to get back in touch with that? What could you see, hear, taste, touch, smell and feel? **(8/12)**

If this doesn't feel good, think of something else. The world's your lobster.

It offers our minds and physiology a little break from all the thinking we can get stuck in. Whatever's going on, we can mentally take ourselves to this happy place or resource. We can reconnect with a sense of peace and safety, happiness and ease.

It can be beneficial before sleeping **(27/1)** or when we feel stressed, overwhelmed and flooded. As with so many tools, the more we practice them when we're ok, the more likely we are to remember them when they'll be especially helpful.

18/12 – Bleed

Having had endometriosis, I've long been aware of the need to rest and sleep more at this time, scheduling lighter days where possible. Lisa Lister's *Code Red* has helped me to reframe this as a time to tap into my intuition and power.

You'll get a clearer idea of what this time of month means for you from cycling **(28/2)**. Many women find this time of month brilliant for prioritising self-care acts like saying 'No' to others' demands, putting your own oxygen mask on first, buying yourself flowers and sleeping in. My symptoms and those of many others are worse during months we haven't, so it's a great incentive for those times we worry about being selfish.

It can be a powerful time for journaling, as intuition can be heightened now - we just need to slow down to pay attention to it. Lister recommends lighting red candles, wearing red lipstick and having a little private altar to honour this time of the cycle.

19/12 – Lotus mud growth

Can you think of a time when something felt impossible and then it was over? You'd survived.

Thinking back to the lotus **(7/7)**, what have you learned from the situation? What advice would you give the younger you **(22/5)** who struggled with some of this journey?

What strengths and transpersonal qualities have you developed as a result?

20/12 – Kintsukori

This Japanese tradition honours the broken places by gracing the rejoined ceramic with gold. Instead of declaring the item damaged beyond repair or desperately trying to conceal the damage, kintsukori acknowledges the damage and points towards post-traumatic growth.

The gold made the broken ceramic even more valuable. It becomes more than it was even if we can't use the vase to hold water anymore.

How might you honour your physical, mental and emotional scars?

21/12 – Yule/Winter Solstice

This ancient festival was adopted by early Christians and evolved into Christmas. It's a great time of year to ponder ways to bring more light and warmth into the days ahead. We can remind ourselves that the darkness and coldness of winter (in the northern hemisphere) need not be scary. New dreams and light can emerge from it.

It's also a great time to release the old and set intentions around the new.

What are you ready to dream into being?

22/12 – Accepting compassion from others

As I learned from Dr Mary Welford in a workshop on Compassion Focused Therapy (www.compassionatemind.co.uk), while self-compassion helps us be more compassionate towards others, we need to open up to receive compassion from others.

Most of these days' ideas are about taking better care of ourselves and knowing there's that knock on effect benefiting others. Today's about accepting and receiving.

Are we better at giving than receiving compassion? How might we open up more to the world around us and the kindness, care and compassion that can come from the world to us?

23/12 – Circles of Concern and Influence

This tool from Stephen Covey's *Seven Habits of Highly Successful People* (Free Press, 1989) can help when we're overwhelmed by stress and worry.

It involves empowering ourselves to both release worries we have no say in while also increasing our influence so we can make a bigger difference in the world.

We might simply write a list of the things we're most concerned about in this moment. Then, we can draw two circles. The large circle represents our current Circle of Concern and the smaller one, inside it, represents our Circle of Influence.

Now we can decide where each of our concerns belongs. Is it something we can influence? The larger our Circle of Influence, the less anxious we're likely to feel. Similarly, by recognising that we can't influence everything, we can maybe let ourselves off certain hooks.

How does your paper look? How might you prefer it to look? What small steps might help you move towards your preferred version?

24/12 – Vision board for the New Year

Vision boards are a great way to keep our dreams at the forefront of our minds. Once we've created something that inspires us (and written 'or something better' somewhere on it), it's helpful to ensure we keep it in mind. I use canvas but we can use any large piece of card or paper. And then we simply cut out images, words and stick them on accordingly. The key is to make it inspiring and uplifting.

Sometimes, we may be unclear on an actual goal and the process of cutting out images and words that speak to us can help us get in touch with a vision. Or we can simply take that pressure off ourselves and call it a mood board. Since seeing Steve Harvey's Oprah interview, I've been taking photos of mine so I can have them as screensavers on my phone and computer.

We can fit it in with our sankalpas **(9/3)** and even bring all the senses online by creating a mood box **(8/12)** specifically for a goal.

25/12 – Christmas

It's been marketed to us since August and is finally here. Whether you have a simple Christmas, enormous extravaganza or don't celebrate at all, what can you do to support yourself through this day that's so laden with expectation?

It may be too late for this year but maybe something unexpected springs to mind. Travelling somewhere else? Volunteering at a shelter? Creating an open house for people without nearby loved ones? Burying your head in a great book and rejoining the world when all the fuss is over?

26/12 – Boxing Day

St Stephen's Day or Boxing Day was apparently a time when people would box up their leftovers for the less fortunate. It's also a time to let the system come down a little after the big lift (and possibly anti-climax) of Christmas. Gatherings tend to be less formal and we may not bother with people at all. What's your idyllic Boxing Day? Does getting in touch with this - however unrealistic - give you any ideas for next year's festive season?

27/12 – Ho'oponopono

This ancient Hawaiian energy clearing system for forgiveness **(9/6)** and reconciliation has been credited with clearing prisons. Because we're all connected, clearing for ourselves has an impact on others. In *Zero Limits*, Joe Vitale (Wiley, 2007) describes all sorts of ways to use it. When I learned about Metta (which also works on the heart's electromagnetic field) **(15/2)**, I was immediately reminded of Ho'oponopono.

It involves a mantra **(23/1)** like meditation: 'I love you, I'm sorry, please forgive me, thank you.'

When I first learned about this, just hearing it described by Dharma Gaynes gave me the chilled feeling of a really good yoga class. I like to use it while swimming. Of course, being human, minds wander but we can bring it back and do our own little bit for peace on earth.

28/12 – What did you love most about this past year?

What stand out as some of your highlights? What and who did you love? When did you feel most relaxed? When were you most inspired? When did you feel most expansive? You get the gist. What stands out for you?

29/12 – Bringing more of what feels best into the year ahead

Having reflected on the year past **(28/12)**, how might you plan to have more of these highlights in the year ahead?

We're not looking to suck the spontaneity and joy from these experiences, just doing more of what feels good more consciously.

Maybe planning to feel better in the year ahead?

30/12 – Preparing to release the past year

In recent years, New Year's Eve for me has become all about letting go, releasing and creating space for a fantabulous new year filled with all good things.

When you think about getting ready to release the heartaches, sorrows and losses from the year just gone, what might help you do so?

I do a major clean*, visualising the past being cleared, cleaned and vacuumed away - and safely released into the earth for recycling - before preparing to contemplate the year ahead.

It's also a great time of year to write letters to not be sent **(1/10)**.

31/12 – Happy New Year!

If you're not a party person, NYE can still have meaning.

Whether I'm going out or not, I write a letter to myself to be read the following NYE. I can't remember who to credit but heard this idea on Hay House Radio years ago. Essentially, the letter contains a list of things I'm grateful for from the year just gone, a list of lessons learned - things that I have reframed into silver linings as well as more joyful lessons - hopes and plans for the future and a thanks in advance. I then pop it into a card, put it away with the Christmas decorations when they all come down and don't revisit it until the following NYE.

This is just one of many things you can play with. You can create your own little rituals to honour the past (and release it) while celebrating the new.

In terms of going out or staying in, how can you make whatever you choose as enjoyable and supportive as possible?

Happy New Year!

---

* some might say I was more fun before I quit alcohol in 2001.

Sources

ANGEL, Elena, www.elenaangel.com.

ASSAGIOLI, Roberto, *The Act of Will,* Penguin, 1977.

BAN BREATHNACH, Sarah, *Simple Abundance,* Bantam, 1997.

BENSON, Herbert, *The Relaxation Response,* Avon Books, 2000.

BERNSTEIN, Gabrielle, *May Cause Miracles,* Hay House, 2013; *The Universe Has Your Back,* Hay House, 2016.

BROWN, Brené, *The Gifts of Imperfection,* Hazelden, 2010; *Rising Strong,* Vermillion, 2015. www.ted.com/talks/brene_brown_on_vulnerability?language=en.

CAIN, Susan, *Quiet,* Penguin, 2012.

CHOQUETTE, Sonia, *Your Three Best Superpowers,* Hay House, 2016; *Trust Your Vibes,* Hay House, 2004.

CLANCE, Pauline, *The Imposter Phenomenon: overcoming the fear that haunts your success,* Peace Tree, 1985; *The Imposter Phenomenon: when success makes you feel like a fake,* Bantam, 1986.

COVEY, Stephen, *Seven Habits of Highly Successful People*, Free Press, 1989.

CUDDY, Amy, *Presence: Bringing your Boldest Self to Your Biggest Challenges,* Little, Brown, 2015. www.ted.com/talks/amy_cuddy_your_body_language_shapes_who_you_are?language=en.

DOWN, Michèle, www.micheledowndynamics.co.uk.

DRAKE, Joy and TYLER, Kathy, angel cards available widely or from Amazon www.amazon.co.uk/Original-Angel-Cards-Book-Inspirational.

DUCKWORTH, Angela, *Grit: The Power of Passion and Perseverance,* Vermillion, 2016.

EMOTO, Masuru, *Message from water and the Universe,* Hay House, 2010.

ENSLER, Eve, *The Vagina Monologues,* Virago, 2001.

FENNINGS-MONKMAN, Gill, www.counsellingforachange.com.

FERRUCCI, Piero, *Inevitable Grace: Breakthroughs in the lives of great men and women: guides to your self-realization,* Tarcher, 2009; *The Power of Kindness,* Penguin, 2006.

FEY, Tina, *Bossy Pants,* Sphere, 2012.

FORD, Debbie, *The Dark Side of the Light Chasers,* Hodder, 2001.

GILBERT, Elizabeth, *Big Magic: creative Living beyond fear,* Bloomsbury, 2015.

GISER, Art, www.energeticnlp.com and www.solar-events.co.uk.

GLENVILLE-CLEAVE, Bridget, *Positive Psychology: A Practical Guide,* Icon Books, 2012.

HALL, Liz, *Mindful Coaching,* Kogan Page, 2013.

HALL, Shaura, www.yogalove.co.uk.

HARRSION, Stephanie, www.lifeguidanceandinspiration.com.

HARVEY, Steve, *Act Like a Success, Think Like a Success,* Amistad, 2015.

JAMES, Tad, www.timelinetherapy.com.

JUDITH, ANODEA, *Chakra Yoga,* Llewellyn Publications, 2015; *Eastern Body, Western Mind,* Celestial Arts, 2004. www.sacredcentres.com.

KATIE, BYRON, *Loving What Is,* Rider, 2002. www.thework.com.

KENNARD, Susan, www.susankennard.co.uk.

KEYES, Marian, *Rachel's Holiday,* Penguin, 1997.

KITCHENER, Lou, www.yogahappy.co.uk.

KONDO, Marie, *Life Changing Magic of Tidying,* Vermillion, 2014.

LAMB, Natalie, nutritionist www.bio-kult.com.

LEVINE, Peter, *Waking the Tiger: Healing Trauma,* North Atlantic Books, 1997.

LISTER, Lisa, *Code Red,* SHE Press, 2015; *Love Your Lady Landscape,* Hay House, 2016. www.thesassyshe.com.

MINVALEEV et al., *Human Physiology,* 2004.

MIRALES, Nancy Jean, www.yourbeautifulchakras.com.

MOHR, Tara, *Playing Big,* Arrow, 2015.

MOOVENTHAN et al, *International Journal of Yoga,* 2014.

MYATT, Clare, www.claremyatt.co.uk.

NORTHRUP, Kate, *Money: A Love Story,* Hay House, 2013.

O'CONNOR, Joseph, *NLP Workbook,* Thorsons, 2001.

POEHLER, Amy, *Yes Please,* Picador, 2015.

REDDY, Jini, *Wild Times,* Bradt, 2016.

RICHARDSON, Cheryl, *The Art of Extreme Self-Care,* Hay House, 2009; *The Unmistakable Touch of Grace,* Bantam, 2005.

ROBERTS, Kath, www.alchemy4thesoul.com.

ROBERTS, Olivia, *Chronic Pain and Debilitating Conditions Resolution*, Findhorn Press, 2012.

ROE, Steve, www.hooplaimpro.com.

ROSENBERG, Marshall, *Nonviolent Communication – A Language of Life,* Puddle Dancer Press, 2015.

ROTHSCHILD, Babette, *The Body Remembers,* WW Norton, 2000.

SANDERSON, Christiane, *The Warrior Within,* One in Four, 2015. www.christianesanderson.co.uk.

SANFILIPPO, Lisa, www.lisayogalondon.com.

SHER, Priya, www.priyasher.com.

STRAYED, Cheryl, *Wild: A Journey from lost to found,* Atlantic Books, 2015.

STREETER, Dr Chris, www.youtube.com/watch?v=asRPQ6m WZUg.

STROZZI Institute, www.strozziinstitute.com.

TAYLOR, Shelly, *Health Psychology,* McGraw Hill, 2011.

TURNBULL, Emma, www.goddessyoga.co.uk.

VITALE, Joe, *Zero Limits*, Wiley, 2007.

WEINTRAUB, Amy, *Yoga for Depression,* Broadway Books, 2004. www.youtube.com/watch?v=_OZ3v3w1h0g.

WELFORD, Mary, *Compassion Focused Therapy for Dummies,* Wiley, 2016; *The Compassionate Mind Approach to Building Self Confidence,* Robinson, 2012. www.compassionatemind.co.uk.

YOUNG, Valerie, *The Secret Thoughts of Successful Women – Why Capable People Suffer from the Imposter Syndrome and How to Thrive in Spite of It*, Crown, 2011.

ZAK, Dr Paul, *The Moral Molecule,* Corgi, 2013.

ZEIDAN et al, *Journal of Neuroscience* and *American Mindfulness Research Monthly.*

ZINN, Jon Kabat, *Full Catastrophe Living,* Piatkus, 2013; *Wherever You Go, There You Are,* Piatkus, 2004.

Index

brahmari 5/4

brain waves 7/4

breath practices (see also pranayama) 7/1, 3/2, 23/2, 29/2, 23/3, 6/5, 29/5

Brown, Brené (shame, vulnerability, wholehearted living) 9/2, 13/2, 27/6, 28/6

Buddha 17/4

Burmese meditation technique 25/3, 13/6

Buttolph, Angela 3/3

C

Cain, Susan 11/10

Cameron, Julia 6/6

Cannon, Walter B 1/1

cardiorespiratory resonance 7/2

Carney, Dana 26/11

Carpenter, Mary 16/4

centring 13/3, 16/11, 27/11

chakra 25/1, 1/2, 6/2, 20/2, 19/3, 20/3, 10/5, 14/5-21/5, 9/7-17/7, 19/7, 29/7, 30/7, 20/8, 29/8, 30/8, 1/9, 4/9-6/9, 9/9, 12/9-13/9, 16/9, 23/9, 29/10

chant 22/1, 23/1, 29/2, 2/3, 5/4, 13/7, 17/7, 18/7

charge 21/1, 25/1, 6/2, 22/3, 4/4, 3/5, 25/6, 30/6, 2/7, 4/7, 16/7, 22/7, 1/8, 9/8

Charmed 27/10

Chekov, Anton 15/4

Chiang, Al Huang 18/4

Child 14/1, 4/3, 22/5, 1/6, 5/6, 8/6, 17/6, 30/6, 18/7, 12/8, 11/10, 28/10, 3/12

Choquette, Sonia 25/2, 16/7

circadian rhythms 29/3

circulation 4/3, 14/3

circulatory system 28/4

Clance, Pauline 12/12

Cognitive Brain Research 9/3

coherent breathing (see also resonant breathing) 7/2, 27/11

colour 9/5-21/5, 3/6, 4/9-10/9, 2/11

compassion 7/1, 10/1, 9/2, 13/2-15/2, 17/2, 20/2, 25/2, 24/3, 17/5-18/5, 22/5, 24/5, 26/5-29/5, 7/6, 13/7, 16/7, 21/8, 30/8, 5/10, 8/10, 22/12

Lehrer, Paul 7/2
Levine, Peter *Waking the Tiger* 14/8
limbic activation 22/1
Lister, Lisa 28/2, 6/3, 25/6, 28/7, 29/9, 8/12
Logical Levels (aka Neurological Levels) 14/10, 17/11-24/11
Loving Kindness (see Metta) 11/2, 15/2, 12/3, 16/3, 13/11
Lughnasadh 1/8
lung capacity 22/1, 22/2, 11/3, 7/4-8/4

M
mantra 5/1, 22/1-23/1, 27/12
Marchetti, Francesca 17/9
McGraw, Dr Phil 8/10
Mead, Margaret 19/4
meditate, meditation, meditative, meditating 1/1, 3/1, 22/1, 5/2, 7/2, 9/2,
    11/2, 15/2, 19/2, 20/3, 26/3-27/3, 4/4-6/4, 13/4, 23/4, 9/5, 20/5, 13/6,
    16/6, 14/7, 21/7, 4/8, 22/8, 27/8-28/8, 2/9, 4/9, 6/9, 14/9, 4/10, 23/10,
    6/11, 14/11, 27/11, 29/11, 2/12, 4/12, 8/12, 17/12, 27/12
menstruation (see also Lisa Lister) 21/2, 28/4-29/4, 28/10
Metta meditations 21/1, 9/2, 11/2, 15/2, 12/3, 16/3, 24/3, 27/9, 27/11,
    27/12
Mime 18/4
mindful, mindfulness 7/1-9/1, 22/1, 5/2, 7/2, 17/2, 22/3-26/3, 3/4, 6/4,
    10/4, 26/4-27/4, 29/5, 8/6, 13/6, 26/6, 1/7, 20/7, 3/8, 5/8-6/8, 16/8, 3/10,
    9/10, 12/10, 15/10
Minvaleev 18/2
Mirales, Nancy Jean 29/10
Mohr, Tara *Playing Big* 25/2
Montgomery, L.M., *Anne of Green Gables* 11/6
Mood box 2/1, 8/12, 24/12
Mooventhan 5/4
Mother Theresa 16/4
mudras 24/4, 3/5-8/5, 9/7, 20/7, 23/7, 29/10, 5/11
Myatt, Clare 1/3, 13/3
Myers, Mike 12/12

N
Native American 5/6, 11/9

neural pathways 3/9, 30/9, 9/10, 9/3

neurotransmitter 30/5, 15/12-16/12

Neuro Linguistic Programming, NLP 3/1, 5/3, 27/3, 8/5, 13/5, 26/5, 29/7, 6/10, 14/10, 3/11, 5/11, 17/11-24/11, 8/12

Nhat Hanh, Thich 26/3

Nightingale, Florence 16/4

Nonviolent Communication, NVC 16/2-17/2

O

Obama, Barack 23/6

O'Connor, Joseph *The NLP Workbook* 13/5

O'Keefe, Georgia 15/4

Om 22/1-23/1, 5/4, 17/7

Ostara/Spring equinox 21/3

oxytocin 2/3, 7/11-8/11, 14/12

P

parasympathetic 1/1, 9/11, 22/1, 26/1, 8/2, 8/3, 3/4, 6/4, 3/10

Patanjali 17/4

Petrarch 15/4

pons 25/11

positive psychology 31/5

power poses 20/2, 30/3, 11/7, 23/7, 6/8, 15/10, 26/11

pranayama, yogic breath practices 7/1, 3/2, 23/2, 7/5, 22/10

  Alternative Nostril Breathing 23/2, 21/3, 7/4, 13/8

  Brahmari 5/4

  belly breath, abdominal breathing 8/1, 29/1-30/1, 3/2, 21/2, 30/4, 2/5, 16/8, 18/8

  Breath of Joy 6/1

  Dirga 8/4

  Kapalabhati 23/2, 22/10

  Ujjayi 7/1, 26/1, 7/2, 23/2, 6/4, 8/4, 30/4, 22/10

  yin breath practice 29/5

prefrontal cortex 7/1, 5/2, 23/5

pregnancy, pregnant 18/2, 23/2, 29/4, 25/6, 25/7, 29/9, 28/10

Psychological Science 27/11

Psychology Today 15/12

psychosynthesis 10/1, 4/2, 25/2, 14/4, 22/5, 31/5, 15/6, 21/8, 21/10, 3/12

Somerstein, Lynne 8/4

Sorkin, Aaron 23/5

space clearing 5/1, 5/3, 18/7, 29/7, 22/8, 27/8, 4/12

Springsteen, Bruce 22/7

St Catherine 20/4

St John of the Cross 20/4

St Teresa 20/4

St Teresa of Avila 17/4

Steinem, Gloria 28/6

Strayed, Cheryl *Wild* 31/7

Streep, Meryl 12/12

Streeter, Dr Chris (working with McLean Hospital's Dr Eric Jensen) 30/5

stress 7/1-8/1, 11/1, 13/1, 6/2, 7/2, 18/2, 20/2-21/2, 26/2, 4/3, 8/3-9/3, 26/3, 3/4, 8/4-9/4, 11/4, 24/4, 9/5, 13/5, 23/5, 25/5-26/5, 30/5, 10/6, 2/7, 18/7, 20/7, 25/7, 11/8-12/8, 15/8, 3/10, 22/10, 26/10, 15/11, 26/11, 3/12, 6/12, 13/12, 17/12, 23/12

Stevens, Philip / Swami Sannyasananda 27/1

Stiles, Mukunda 28/10

subpersonalities, subpersonality 10/1-19/1, 3/3, 16/3, 18/4, 3/10, 20/10, 14/11

suicide 10/9

Summer Solstice (also Litha) 21/6

Suzuki, Sunryu 17/4

Swift, Taylor 3/11

sympathovagal balance 7/2

T

Tai Chi 18/4

tarot 19/2, 31/8

Taylor, Shelly 3/10

Telles, Shelly 22/1

telomeres 4/8

tend and befriend 3/10

testosterone 18/2, 25/6, 29/9, 26/11

Thropp, Elphaba (*Wicked*) 28/4, 12/5

Timeline Therapy 20/1-21/1

Tolstoy 17/4

transference 10/4

Social intelligence 31/5, 22/6
Spirituality 31/5, 23/11, 7/12
Vitality 31/5, 6/12
Wisdom 5/1, 19/1, 1/2, 15/2, 25/2, 1/3, 9/3, 17/3, 27/3, 19/5-20/5, 29/5,
   31/5, 14/7-15/7, 24/7, 29/7, 24/8, 28/8-29/8, 11/9, 23/9, 10/10, 15/10,
   26/10-27/10, 31/10

V
vagus and vagal tone 23/2, 29/2, 6/4, 30/4, 22/10
Van Gogh, Vincent 15/4
vestibular system 30/3, 16/11
vision board 5/1, 25/6, 13/10, 24/12
Vitale, Joe 27/12

W
Walker, Alice 20/6
Walsh, Peter 19/3
Walter, Dawna 19/3
The Ways 14/4-21/4
Weintraub, Amy, *Yoga for Depression* 6/1
Welford, Dr Mary 22/12
well-formed outcomes 6/10-9/10, 13/10, 17/11
The Will 15/6-16/6, 3/12
   Good Will 15/6
   Skilful Will 15/6
   Strong Will 15/6
   Transpersonal Will 15/6
Williamson, Marianne 27/3
willpower 12/4, 14/10, 15/12
Wilmot, Joan 8/12
Winfrey, Oprah 19/3, 3/6, 23/6, 6/7, 4/10, 24/12
Winslet, Kate 12/12
Wong, YJ 10/6
Wood Brooks, Allison *Get Excited: Reappraising pre-performance
   anxiety as excitement* 22/7
Wordsworth, William 15/4

Y

Yap, Andy 26/11

Yang, YC et al. 19/8

Yin breath practice 29/5

yoga 3/1-4/1, 6/1-7/1, 23/1-24/1, 27/1-31/1, 1/2, 6/2-7/2, 10/2-11/2, 15/2, 18/2, 20/2-21/2, 26/2-27/2, 29/2, 8/3-9/3, 14/3, 16/3, 18/3, 24/3, 30/3-31/3, 3/4, 5/4-6/4, 16/4, 18/4, 23/4, 28/4-30/4, 3/5, 30/5, 13/6, 16/6, 10/7-12/7, 14/7-16/7, 21/7, 24/7, 4/8, 6/8, 15/8-16/8, 20/8, 17/10, 22/10, 26/10, 28/10, 4/11, 6/11-7/11, 15/11-16/11, 25/11, 8/12, 15/12, 17/12, 27/12

backbends 10/2-11/2, 21/2, 14/3, 27/7, 18/8, 15/11

Bow 21/2, 10/7

Bridge (also Little Bridge) 11/3, 14/3, 15/11

Camel 12/7, 27/7

Cat/Cow 30/4, 10/7, 16/8-17/8

Chair 18/3, 3/4, 11/4, 15/11

Child 4/3, 1/6, 16/6, 28/10

Cow Faced pose 12/7, 26/7

Down Dog, Downward Facing Dog 22/2, 28/4, 30/4

Fish 12/7-13/7

Handstand 28/4, 2/6

Hare 15/7, 28/7

Headstand 28/4, 15/7

Inversions 28/4-29/4

Legs up Against the Wall 28/4-29/4, 2/5

Lunge 11/4

Lion 4/3

Mini Cobra 18/2

Mountain 9/7, 16/11

Pigeon 10/7, 18/8, 15/11

Plough 2/5, 25/7

Prayer position 24/4

Restorative Fish 23/1, 11/2, 15/2, 12/7-13/7

Savasana 22/10, 26/10

Seated Forward Fold 17/3, 31/3

Seated Twist 31/1, 11/7

Shoulder Stand 1/5-2/5, 13/7, 25/7

Simple Twist 30/1